I0104072

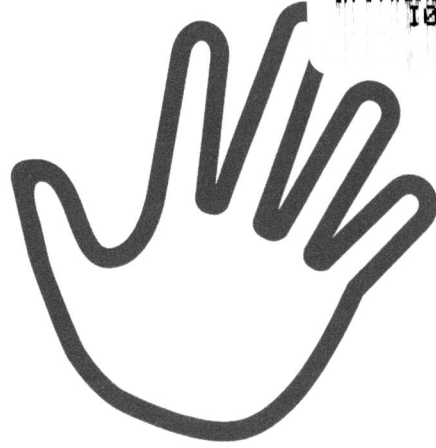

101 WAYS TO IMPROVE YOUR HEALTH WITH BODY WORK

Your Complete Guide to Complementary and Alternative Therapies

ALAN E. SMITH

Loving Healing Press

Ann Arbor, MI

101 Ways to Improve Your Health with Body Work: Your Complete Guide to Complementary & Alternative Therapies.
Copyright © 2017 Alan E. Smith, All Rights Reserved.

No part of this publication may be reproduced, transmitted in any form or by any means, electronic, mechanical, photocopying, recording, or other otherwise, or stored in a retrieval system, without the prior written consent of the author or publisher.

Learn more about this subject and listen to our free podcasts at
www.UnBreakYourHealth.com

Library of Congress Cataloging-in-Publication Data

Names: Smith, Alan E., 1951- author.
Title: 101 ways to improve your health with body work : your complete guide
  to complementary & alternative therapies / by Alan E. Smith.
Other titles: One hundred one ways to improve your health with body work
Description: Ann Arbor, MI : Loving Healing Press, [2017] | Includes index.
Identifiers: LCCN 2017002395 (print) | LCCN 2017005779 (ebook) | ISBN
  9781615993338 (pbk. : alk. paper) | ISBN 9781615993345 (ebk) | ISBN
  9781615993345 (ePub, PDF, Kindle)
Subjects: LCSH: Alternative medicine--Popular works. | Mind and body
  therapies--Popular works. | Self-care, Health--Popular works.
Classification: LCC R733 .S618 2017 (print) | LCC R733 (ebook) | DDC 613--dc23
LC record available at https://lccn.loc.gov/2017002395
Distributed by: Ingram Book Group, New Leaf Distributing, and Bertram's Books (UK)

Published by:
Loving Healing Press
5145 Pontiac Trail
Ann Arbor, MI 48105
USA

www.LovingHealing.com or
info@LovingHealing.com
Fax 734-663-6861
TollFree 888-761-6268

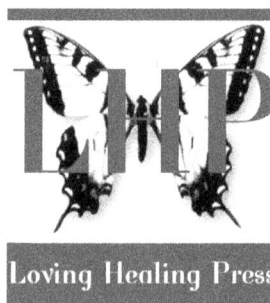
Loving Healing Press

CONTENTS

Disclaimer

This book is not intended to diagnose or prescribe any treatment for any medical or psychological condition(s), nor does it claim to prevent, diagnose, treat, mitigate, or cure any medical or psychological conditions.

It contains the ideas and opinions of its author and is intended solely to provide helpful information on a variety of subjects. It is sold with the understanding that the author and publisher are not engaged in rendering medical, health or any other kind of personal professional services in the book.

The reader should consult his or her medical, health or other competent professional before adopting any of the suggestions in the book.

The author and publisher specifically disclaim all responsibility for any liability, loss, or risk, personal or otherwise, that is incurred as a consequence (directly or indirectly) of the use and application of any of the contents of this book.

Introduction

This book is all about hope. From ancient healing therapies to the latest American innovations, you have more options for great health today than ever before. Complementary and alternative therapies, known as CAM, are about more than just improving your health. These therapies are about helping you rediscover the joy, the wonder and the beauty of living.

Perhaps the aches and pains that caused you to stumble are caused from your body being out of alignment in some way so it's a body issue. Maybe an emotional issue or traumatic life experience is seeking resolution by expressing itself through the body, so it could be a mind issue. Or your life force energy could be blocked in some way resulting in a physical problem so it could be a spirit or energy issue.

In this guide you'll find information new and old and begin to see patterns between therapies that are consistent through thousands of years and across civilizations around the world.

The most basic concept is that you are the sum of your Mind-Body-Spirit. Your parts cannot be disconnected so a problem in one area can mean problems in all areas. Holistic (or whole-istic) therapies are effective because they address all of you. Many of these complementary and alternative therapies work to prevent problems or correct them as soon as possible to prevent them from growing into serious issues. This is a very different approach from medicine in America today which is based on fee-for-service.

Once you start talking with friends and family about these new options it seems like everybody knows somebody who's experienced success, sometimes miraculous success, with a complementary or alternative therapy. While writing this book, I've been amazed at the stories from friends and yet we still seem to talk about CAM in whispers, as if it's something normal people don't discuss in public. I hope this book brings complementary and alternative therapies out of the shadows and into the light of day so more people can discover a healthier, happier new life.

According to the 2007 NCCAM report on complementary and alternative medicine 38% of Americans used some form during the previous 12 months. This is a dramatic change from the 62% reported in the 2002 study but that's because the government studies dropped the use of prayer as a form of CAM. Apparently the use of this ancient, some say the original, energy therapy was too popular to be included in the study because it skewed the data making it appear that CAM was too popular.

The data in the federal government reports is from the National Health Interview Survey conducted by the U. S. Department of Health & Human Services, the Center for Disease Control's National Center for Health Statistics. For the 2007 report, NHIS interviews were completed in 29,266 households, which yielded 75,764 persons in 29,915 families and a household response rate of 87.1%. Between the 2002 and 2007 government reports acupuncture, deep breathing exercises, massage therapy, meditation, naturopathy, and yoga showed significant increases.

Perhaps one of the reasons for the explosive growth and popularity of complementary and alternative therapies is the fact that people appreciate being much more than just a number on a form. Every person is a unique individual composed of mind, body and spirit (or life-force energy). All facets must be healthy and balanced for wellness and personal growth. A PBS-TV special in 2006 featured doctors talking about their hope for the trend in medicine to go back to treating patients as whole beings. Many of them wondered how Western medicine could have ever gotten so far off track to ignore the mind and spiritual components of every patient in the first place.

Complementary and alternative therapies also focus on individualized treatments, rather than assembly-line, one-size-fits-all medicine. Every person and their health problems are unique, usually resulting from a combination of factors. These therapies tend to look at the whole person for the source of the problem, not just the symptoms that bring them in the door.

In this era of entitlement, too many people have come to believe they are owed good health and this has led to a passive national attitude towards health. When we get sick, we expect the doctor to give us a pill, a shot or perform some surgery to fix us right up so we can continue living without having to make any changes in our lives or accept responsibility for our own health.

One of the major themes of complementary and alternative therapies is personal responsibility. Who better to take care of *your* body than YOU? After all, who has more "skin in the game" of your life than you do? These complementary and alternative therapies offer new and old ways for better health but you, the person reading this book, will have to care enough about your life to take personal responsibility for your health. Empowering yourself with information about all of the health care options available today is the first step in order for you to make the most informed decisions possible about your health care.

Another difference between standard medicine and CAM today is a focus on wellness and the ingredients for health. Among other things, we need proper diet, exercise and a way to release the stress of the day. You've probably already heard these recommendations from medical doctors. These aren't new ideas; in fact they're very old. Four hundred years ago Jonathan Swift, author of *Gulliver's Travels*, said that "The best doctors in the world are Doctor Diet, Doctor Quiet and Doctor Merryman." Today, four centuries later we're still discovering the importance to our health today of what we eat and drink, the peace that we find within ourselves and the joy that we find in life. Sad to admit but we usually take better care of our cars and our yards than we do our most precious gift, our own health.

America has neglected complementary and alternative therapies in favor of scientific Western medicine for over 100 years. While this profit-driven orientation has produced some outstanding developments, much has also been sacrificed. Today, the newest scientific equipment is confirming that we are all *whole beings* of mind, body and spirit, often raising more questions than providing answers. The explosion of research in neuroscience is changing the meaning of the expression "It's all in your head" because technology is showing how the mind is related to and controls the body. We're moving quickly from simple correlation of the mind-body connection to discovering the actual mechanisms of interaction. Epigenetics is showing us how the power of our own thoughts and feelings can change the functioning of our genes.

Because so many of these complementary and alternative therapies are based on a completely different paradigm (energy) they operate on different principles than the standard chemical model of the human body. This means they can't be studied using the same methodology as current research. They also function as whole systems and cannot be examined piece by piece. Using existing research models for CAM is simply like trying to put a square peg in a round hole. Much like quantum physics, the very act of observation influences the results. Even the White House Commission on Complementary and Alternative Medicine Policy understood this concept. The 2002 report said "Research is needed to pursue answers to questions posed by CAM that lie outside the conventional medical paradigm."

Everything in this book will work for someone, but nothing in this book will work for everyone. The same is true with mainstream medicine. Some pills help people while the same medication may be ineffective or even harmful to someone else. There is a wide variety in the quality of medical doctors and it's the same with the practitioners of these healing arts. Whether it's a medical doctor or an alternative practitioner you should always research their qualifications and training and then enter into any relationship with an attitude of Buyer Beware. Remember, you are in charge of your health! Just as it's always been recommended to seek out second opinions for diagnosis by a medical doctor, practicing the same approach would be beneficial when working with complementary or alternative therapies too.

Not every type of CAM will be found in this book. Quite frankly, some are practiced by only a few people while others are being created so quickly that it's almost impossible to keep track. Being human, it's possible my research has missed some valuable therapies. Some of the therapies listed are FDA approved but because they're still ignored by most doctors, they're still considered outside of the "norm".

Rather than trying to swamp you with all types of therapies I've broken my research down into three separate books. This edition focuses on all of the Body Therapies or the physical aspect of your health. While I've added listings from my last guide the nature of CAM means it will never be complete because innovation is constantly adding new therapies and techniques. If you don't feel an urge to explore one of these treatments then perhaps the answer to your health concerns will be in the Mind Therapies or Energy/Spirit Therapies editions.

What started out as a quest to improve my own Baby Boomer health has resulted in this collection of information and opportunities. Like so many people, conventional medicine ran out of ideas to help me, so I had to start looking for new options and fortunately I've found them. Researching this book has been an enjoyable and enlightening adventure. It's also testimony to the fact that there is hope: you can find your own answers just as I have.

This reference guide to complementary and alternative therapies is the result of research and interpretation of each modality, or type of process. In many cases there are a variety of opinions, so please remember this is simply *one* opinion. With the steady stream of innovation happening today this volume is not intended as a finished work but simply a starting place for your quest for better health and a better life, which is why so many websites are included to help your quest.

Readers who also enjoy listening to learn more about complementary and alternative therapies will enjoy *UnBreak Your Health - The Podcast* on our website at www.unbreakyourhealth.com. We've built a library of 20-minute podcast interviews featuring the leading authorities in America discussing their therapy. Whenever you see the podcast microphone listed, it means there is a podcast on that subject available.

You're going to be amazed to discover the variety of complementary and alternative therapies available today, and how effective they can be. The hope you've been looking for to improve your health is right here.

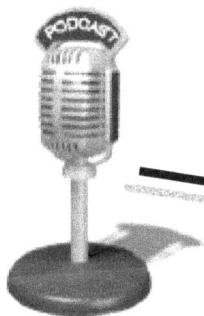

This icon means there's an interview with one of the leading authorities on this therapy at www.UnbreakYourHealth.com/podcasts.htm

Chapter 1 - Your Map to Better Health

I met Karen after one of my speeches. She was in her early 50s and in generally good health but with a few chronic problems the doctors just couldn't seem to get a handle on, frustrating both her and them. One doctor had told her to "just learn to live with it" and simply walked out of the examining room in a rush to his next patient. I told her I knew exactly how she felt because I'd been there too. When the doctor says there's nothing more he can do for you, it's a very lonely, even scary, place to be. Where do you go now? What can you do?

She was resigned to her health problems but still held on to a thread of hope, one that she was eager to grow into a rope so she could climb out of that unhappy place and into a healthy life. I told Karen that I'd learned that just because doctors can't do anything, that doesn't mean there isn't anything left to do! There are literally hundreds of complementary and alternative therapies available today that have been proven safe and effective for decades, hundreds, even thousands of years. She smiled.

She began to tell me her symptoms expecting that I could instantly tell her which therapy would work best for her condition. I explained to her that I could show her the map of my path to better health but she would have to find her own path because she was a unique and very special human being, different from me and everyone else on the planet.

I added that finding the real source of our health problems is the first step and it's different for every person. Using an example from my radio appearances I told her that if there are three people in the doctor's office with allergy problems they may each have a different source of their health problem. While the doctor may prescribe the same drugs to treat their symptoms it wouldn't deal with the source of their health problem.

Let's say the first person is a hard-working guy in jeans, flannel shirt and boots and his allergy problem may, in fact, originate in his body. In his case a therapy like NAET would be best because it's based on chiropractic and acupressure principles so it's a body-type of treatment.

But the second person is a petite woman in a stylish, professional outfit and the source of her allergy is in her subconscious. That means a Body therapy wouldn't do her any good at all. Because I'm a former PSYCH-K practitioner I told Karen about a client of mine, a woman who would get severe migraines every time she ate Mexican food, to illustrate the problem. Using PSYCH-K we discovered a relationship she'd had with a Mexican boy more than 10 years earlier was the source of her food "allergy" and with a few balances we corrected the problem. Today she eats Mexican food without any headache at all!

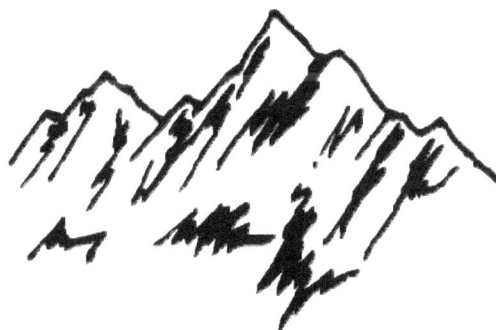

However the third person with an allergy problem is a young man, a student, and the source of his problem isn't in his body or his mind, it's in his energy system/spirit, so a body or mind therapy wouldn't help him. He would need acupuncture, EFT or some type of energy therapy to solve his problem.

Karen looked at me with surprise, you could almost

see the light bulb go on above her head. "I've never heard illness described that way but it makes so much sense!" she said. "Now that I have a better idea of what I'm looking for I can begin to imagine myself finally getting better health."

She spoke with both understanding and yet uncertainty, unsure of what her next step should be. What could or should she do, how could she find her path to better health? I offered her a blank piece of paper and told her this was the beginning of her very own map to better health. With a frown she protested that there was nothing on it. I agreed but explained that's because she had always relied on others for her health. She would fill in her own map as she discovered the truth about her health, her life and her own unique path to better health. By reading her way through this book and others she would learn all about the features of her own life and what benefits different therapies had to offer her, a necessary first step to finding out where you want to go. She would discover for herself what would work and also what wasn't very effective. In other words, she would draw her own map in the colors of her life and find her own unique path. Once again, she smiled with understanding.

I wrote this book just as if I were talking with Karen about how to find her own map to better health. Just imagine that all of these therapy listings are like newspaper clippings, magazine articles and notes from a friend to help you, along with a few comments and suggestions of course! Because I've been the one sitting in the doctor's office after being told there's nothing more mainstream medicine can do to help I wrote a book so others would have a map to find hope. Now I know there is *always* hope.

There's an old saying that religions are just different paths up the mountain to the same destination. In many ways the different types of treatments and therapies available today are like different paths up the mountain of your life to the pinnacle of health. Some paths may be smooth and easy while others may be rocky and challenging (but possibly more rewarding). Perhaps one path is a straight line for a particular health problem, other times that particular path may become winding and indirect. The most important thing to remember is that no matter which path you choose, you are the only one who can walk it. Nobody can live your life for you and no one else can walk your path to better health. We each enjoy a unique life.

Like Karen, you were probably hoping for a nice American-style book where you can just look up your condition or disease and find all of the complementary and alternative therapies for it. Sorry, but as I explained to her sitting in a corner of the meeting room that afternoon, that's not how your health works and it's not how most CAM therapies work either.

In order to unbreak your health you're going to have to find the path that works for you. Before we had satellite-based GPS navigation systems people used maps to help them find their way. For thousands of years we figured out where we were, where we wanted to go and the best way to get there with paper maps. From flat to folded, from simple to full-color, civilization moved forward with maps. However to use a map effectively requires an understanding of its elements and how they must all work together to be useful.

Did you know that paper maps are better for you than GPS systems? You've probably heard news reports of crashes caused by GPS navigation but they've caused other problems like having a house in Atlanta demolished by mistake. It turns out our brains need the mental exercise of maps. In London, one of the most confusing cities in the world, cabbies spend two to four years learning "The Knowledge" of the city before they can start driving. Tests have shown the hippocampus in the brain of these cabbies is substantially larger than the average population. Scientists are concerned that reliance on GPS may even cause earlier onset of dementia in the years to come because we simply aren't exercising our brains with maps.

We learn to navigate with maps using either a spatial strategy that involves learning relationships between various landmarks or the stimulus- response approach that encodes specific routes by memorizing a series of cues. If you have no sense of direction you may suffer from developmental topographical disorientation or DTD. The good news: it can get better with practice. So even though you may not know your way around the world of complementary and alternative medicine now, reading this book will help you learn and find your way.

This book can be your map to better health. There are going to be 3 books, each one focusing on a single area - Body, Mind and Energy/Spirit - corresponding to the functions of a map. This is the Body book which represents the physical world, the landscape of our lives. There are rivers and mountains, plains and plateaus, terrain that presents different degrees of difficulty. Finding your best path requires recognition of these challenges and their opportunities.

The Mind book corresponds to the man-made order we create to better understand the world around us. We created longitude and latitude, name countries and cities; we live in a world of artificial labels developed to help us navigate through life.

The Energy/Spirit book deals with the unseen world of magical energy. Is it really so different from the "magic" that makes a compass work? The unseen force of magnetism makes a compass point North so we can determine which direction we should go to reach our destination. There are magical energies our science is just beginning to understand that can help us find our way to better health.

To use a map effectively you need all of these features to determine where you are, where you want to go, and the best way to get there. Finding better health is your most important journey and this book is one step to help you find your way. To accomplish your goal you'll need to recognize the landscape features that shape and color your world, the mental creations that identify your world, and finding your own compass to discover which direction you're headed. Finding better health also usually requires unlocking the unlimited healing potential of the Body, the Mind and Energy/Spirit.

You are responsible for your own health because no one else has as much to gain or lose from your health as you do. You can't blame your doctor, or your parents, or anybody else. It's your life and you choose to live it the way you want every day. You make the choices that produce the health you have right now. Did you choose a path for long health with good diet, daily exercise habits and deep religious convictions or regular meditation? Or did you choose to eat fast food and put off worrying about your health until later (probably until something breaks)? Taking personal responsibility for your own health is the first step towards finding your path, you're opening your own map. Next you have to empower yourself with knowledge so you can make the most informed decisions possible about your health care and that includes all of your options, even the world of complementary and alternative therapies.

You have many different pathways to choose from for your health and you're the one with the ultimate responsibility of choice. For one health problem you may choose mainstream (allopathic) medicine. For a different health problem you may choose some type of complementary or alternative therapy (CAM). Your constantly changing health may require you to change direction depending on the changing terrain of your condition. You can even walk with a foot on different healing pathways to reach your destination. For example you can add a complementary therapy path alongside the steps you're taking with mainstream medicine. The good news is you have free will and can choose whichever path you want at any time, changing direction as you desire.

One possible path you can choose is standard Western medicine, a popular choice for Americans because it also involves the least amount of personal responsibility and the largest amount of insurance coverage. Here the symptoms of your health problem will be taken care of with prescription drugs or surgery and you're back to your old life. For many this is the tollway of health: fast and easy but expensive. (Fortunately for most people the human body has unlimited healing abilities.)

Other times the path of mainstream medicine may be more complicated, requiring you to go from specialist to specialist to specialist. When that happens this path can turn scary, strange and dark as you try to feel your way around without adequate information. Too often the current medical system fails to treat patients as people, but instead simply a number on a form.

This path can even become quite rocky if you try to share it with some type of complementary or alternative therapy. Most doctors are given little, if any, education in CAM and virtually no training. Doctors do not need any education in complementary and alternative medicine to get a medical license in America today. Most of us fear and dislike what we don't know, regardless of its benefit, so it's no surprise that doctors usually discourage patients from straying from the path of Western medicine. You should always talk with your doctor about your involvement with any type of CAM so he's aware of your complete health situation, but don't expect a sympathetic or even informed response.

A nearby path is called Integrative Medicine, a new type of medicine that tries to capitalize on some of the CAM therapies to find the best solution for an individual's health problem. These doctors are promoting an integrated model of health care in America that incorporates body, mind and spirit. These progressive folks realize that Western medicine doesn't have all of the answers to our health problems today. In general Integrative Medicine doctors are much more open to discussing CAM options even if it's outside their scope of experience. Currently there are 44 member organizations of the Consortium of Academic Health Centers for Integrative Medicine leading the way for better health in this country.

There are also paths that involve what I consider crossover therapies like Osteopathy, a unique American medical innovation. In my podcast interview with Dr. Philip Slocum, the Dean of the Kirksville College of Osteopathic Medicine at A. T. Still University, we talked about how D.O.'s treat the whole patient instead of looking at them as simply a series of systems to be fixed. Osteopaths are fully-trained medical doctors with additional specialized education and training in the body's neuromuscular-skeletal system. Manipulation of this connected system to permit the body to function correctly is critical for the body to heal itself. *(Dr. A. T. Still developed Osteopathy and opened the first college of its kind in the world. Podcast interviews on this and many other therapies can be found at www.unbreakyourhealth.com.)*

One of the first things you'll notice that's different about pathways for complementary and alternative medicine is that they're for all of you, not just for one part or symptom of you. These therapies recognize that you're a unique individual of mind, body and spirit and every health problem is going to involve all of you. CAM therapies also look for the real source of your health problem instead of simply treating symptoms; they have a different perspective about your health.

Do you remember the old joke about the three blind mice and the elephant? One mouse is holding on to the tail and says "An elephant is long and skinny with hair on the end." The next mouse is touching the leg and he says, "No, an elephant is big and round." The third mouse is on the trunk and he says, "You're both wrong. It's not too thick or too thin, but watch out for all of the hot air!" It's similar when you're trying to figure out what's causing your pain or health problem; you need to look at your whole being for the source of your problem rather than just dealing with the individual symptoms.

Just because you may have a name for your condition doesn't mean it's the source of your problem, you have to see the whole elephant. Let me give you an example: let's say you have a pain in your shoulder so you go to your friendly allopathic (mainstream) medical doctor. He checks it out and finds there is nothing broken or torn so he gives you a drug for pain, maybe one for muscle relaxation and possibly another drug to reduce inflammation. (Remember the problems caused by Vioxx?) This is simply to mask the uncomfortable symptoms while your body (hopefully) heals itself.

A practitioner of a complementary or alternative therapy is usually going to look at you as a whole system to see what's causing the problem. Perhaps you're moving the shoulder in an awkward manner which is causing the strain and pain. A Rolfer or Feldenkrais practitioner is going to realign your body so it moves correctly, removing the strain which eliminates the pain without drugs. *(There are free podcast shows on Rolfing and the Feldenkrais Method too at unbreakyourhealth.com.)*

Or perhaps there is a problem with an organ or body function that has changed your body's energy system causing the muscles to tighten in an unusual way which puts a strain on the body. A therapy like acupuncture, EFT or BodyTalk would realign your body's energy flow allowing the body to repair the problem.

The Alexander Method would teach you how to move with efficiency to prevent the wear and tear and pain. Or perhaps it's stress that's literally beating you down and putting your body into awkward positions. Tai Chi, yoga or meditation would help relieve the stress before it produces a physical problem like hunching your shoulders into a painful position. (Doctors now say that up to 80% of our physical problems could actually be stress-related.)

An example of finding the source of a health problem comes from my own life and it involves Rolf Structural Integration therapy. A few years ago I hurt my back doing yard work and when my chiropractor couldn't resolve the situation I decided to try Rolfing. As one of the structural integration therapies the first thing the practitioner had me do was walk back and forth so she could see how my body moved as a whole. The first thing she said was that I must have terrible pain in my knees. I explained to her I'd had pain so bad for over twenty years that at times I couldn't even walk across our local mall. I'd been to orthopedic specialists, neurology specialists ... I'd been all up and down the alphabet of medical specialties looking for help. The only one who did me any good was a podiatrist who sold me an expensive set of custom orthopedic inserts which helped with the symptoms but didn't solve the problem.

The Rolf therapist just waved her hand as if to say "don't worry about it, we'll take care of it" which I found amazing. Now Rolfing began with their Basic Ten series of treatments and true to her word after the third session I took the insoles out of my shoes and haven't worn them since. Today I'm able to hit a treadmill without pain thanks to finding the source of my problem.

This is just an example of how CAM therapies treat the source of the problem, not just the symptoms. Practitioners of complementary and alternative therapies look at the whole person to find what's wrong so they can correct the problem where it begins rather than where it ends. There are many paths to choose from but you're the one responsible for finding the right one (therapy) for your unique health problem. No one else can do it for you any more than someone else can eat your dinner for you. You're the only one who knows what feels right and what doesn't, what makes sense to you for your situation.

This book looks at just one type of CAM therapies: Body. After careful consideration, each subject is classified based on my opinion regarding the primary goal or operating principle. For example, some Energy Medicine can be found in the Body section. This subject is based on the incredible discovery by Dr. Bjorn Nordenstrom of a new circulatory system in the human body for electrical energy called the Biological Closed Energy Circuit (BCEC). Since it deals with the physical system of moving energy through the body it's classified as a physical subject although it deals with the body's energy system, which some consider a spiritual life force.

Acupuncture, on the other hand, is found in the book featuring Energy/Spirit even though it also deals with the body's energy system. Developed 5,000 years ago the ancient Chinese called this energy Chi, or life force. They described it as being a balance of Yin and Yang forces in the body, while Dr. Nordenstrom calls it positive and negative ions of electrical energy. These two listings may, in fact, be talking about the same system but they're classified into two different categories based upon my opinion of their focus or intention.

In an effort to help understand each subject as well as possible similarities to other therapies I often include a little history or perspective with a description of each listing. As you read through this book you'll begin to see many common features and concepts.

User Comments have been included at the end of many listings for a better understanding of each therapy. These are anonymous comments from people who've actually experienced the process. Comments from different people are marked with a diamond-shaped bullet. These testimonials have been collected from a variety of sources to give you a more personal perspective on each therapy. Please remember results are unique to each individual. Because of our uniqueness a process that works well for one person may perform very differently for another. This feature will at least provide a little human color to the black-and-white definitions and descriptions.

Most listings offer websites for you to begin your own research into selected processes. Remember these are just a place to begin your own process of exploration, there are many websites available.

This book is a map to begin your journey to health and happiness, not a quick fix. You'll have to read the whole map to figure out where you are, where you've been, and where you want to go. Only then can you determine the best path to reach your destination given the terrain, roadways, etc. Even if you're just looking for shortcuts you'll want to know all of your options in order to choose the best shortcut. Reading this whole book on Body Therapies will be the first step in taking responsibility for your health.

So how do you unbreak your health and restore its original condition or better? You take responsibility for your own health and take careful steps to improve it by the path you select with each day. You create your own map to better health one step at a time with the choices you make. Starting with a blank page, you fill it in with your own experiences, good and bad. Step by step you'll recognize what helps and what you should avoid. It's nothing new really because you've taken prescription drugs that had side effects you didn't like and drugs that simply didn't work but you kept trying until you find what worked for you. Now we're going to do the same thing with more natural, holistic therapies so you can find a better way to health.

When meeting with any type of healthcare practitioner remember to take your common sense and intuition. Ask questions, lots and lots of questions, because empowerment is the key to understanding your personal map to better health. Remember, it's your life we're talking about!

Please read this book with an open mind and pay attention to your big picture of health, not just to find a magic bullet answer to your current health problems. All of this information will filter deep into your mind and you'll discover that you're naturally drawn to certain subjects. Just as I've discovered new ways to better health, so can you. Welcome to the map to find hope, the path to better health

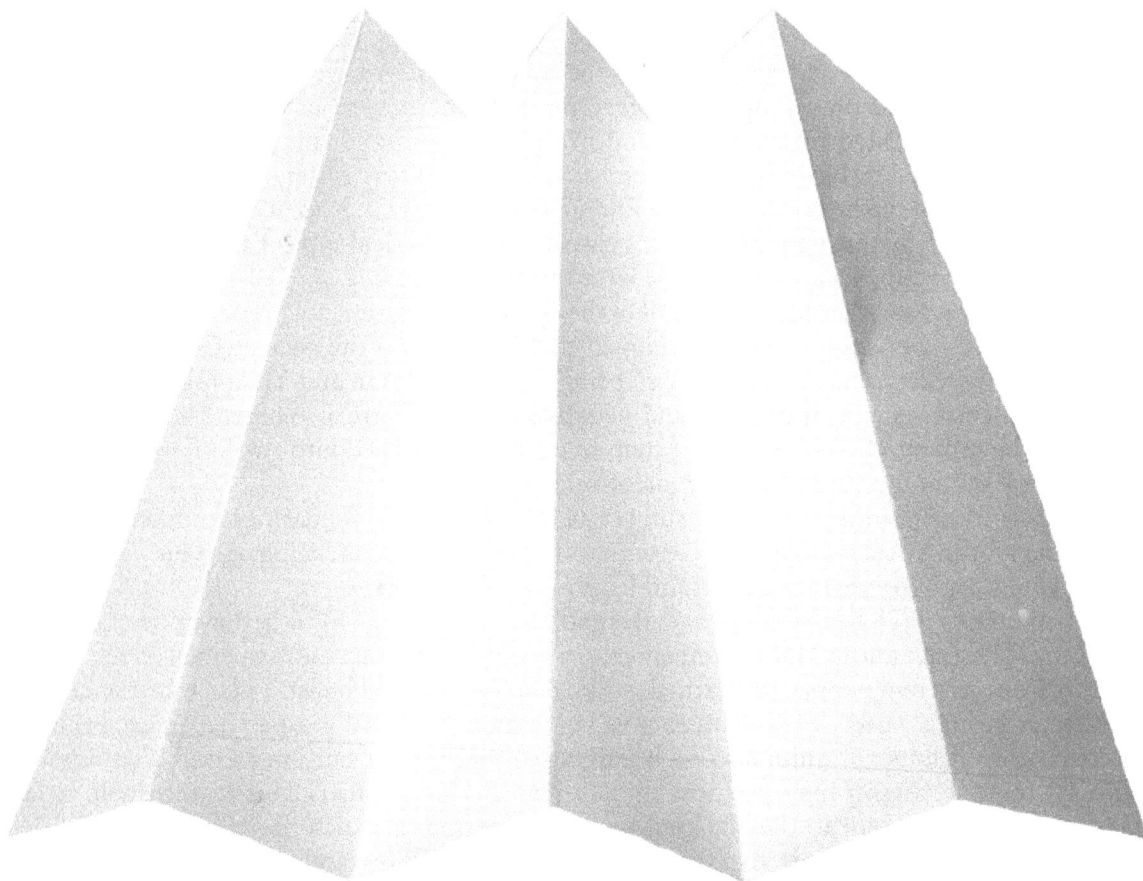

Chapter 2 – The Physical Landscape

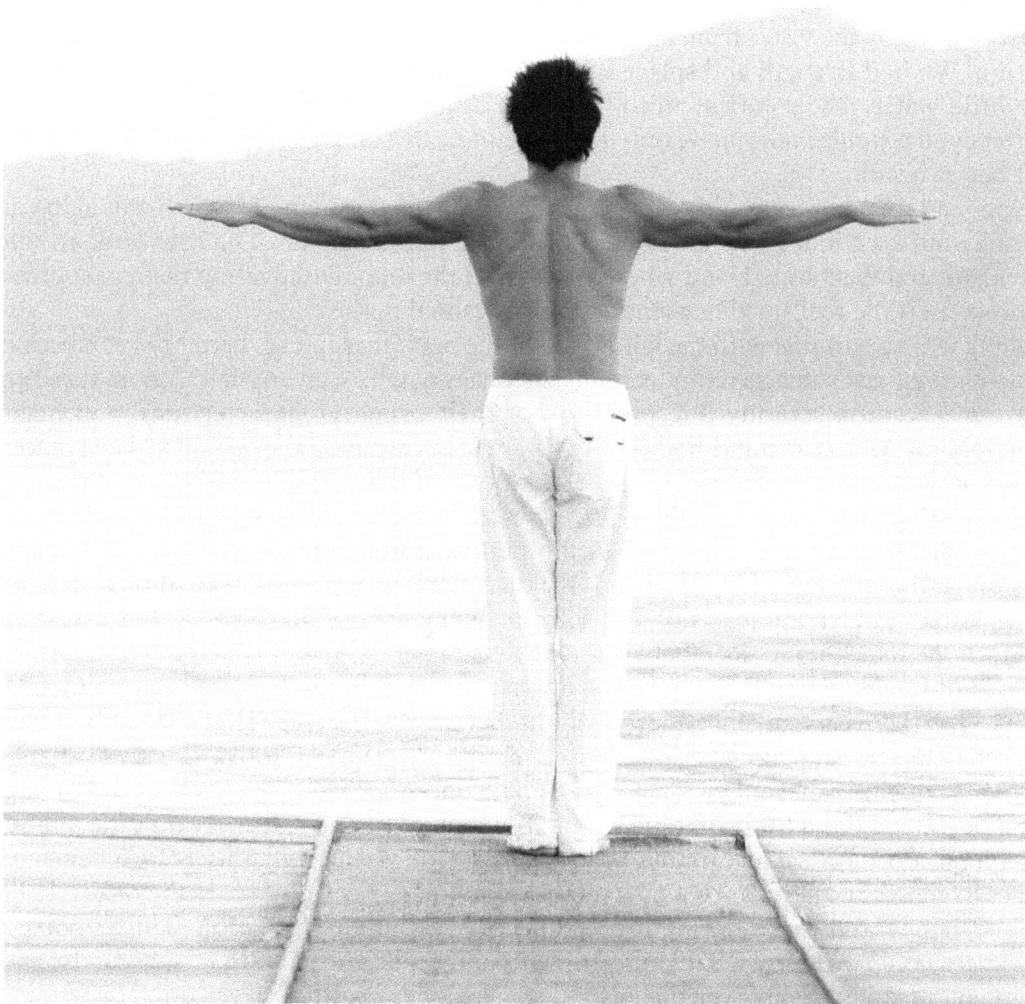

Introduction to Body Category

If you're the kind of person who wants better health then this is the place to start your quest. If you've only experienced mainstream medicine before then you're going to be delighted with the results you discover from the world of complementary and alternative medicine.

We'll begin your exploration into this amazing new world of opportunities for health with the body category. Remember to think of these therapy listings as if they were newspaper clippings, magazine articles and such that a good friend might give you to help with your health problems. Of course there will also be a few words of advice along the way.

Most of us enjoy the vistas from a mountain top or seashore, the view all the way to the horizon is inspiring. We find strength and solace in these places, as if we somehow see how we fit into the world a little better. The colors seem to be a little brighter, the details a little sharper to us. This book offers you a similar new view, only this time of health and healing. It will help you find your place of better health.

As you read this chapter you'll recognize landmarks in your own life which will help you better understand your own map. Just like the old-fashioned paper maps you have to look around to see where you are and then understand where you are on the map. Discovering the real source of your health problem is the real starting point on your personal map.

In many ways beginning with the landscape of the body therapies is better for you because these are some of the easiest subjects to understand since they can be seen and felt. Again, these processes are organized according to my interpretation of their primary characteristics, you may have a different opinion. Many are mind-body-energy techniques meaning they could've been placed just as easily into other books.

It's interesting that so many of these processes are popular with entertainers and athletes since their bodies are strained day after day during performances and competitions. Their livelihood depends on getting the most from their body with minimum wear and tear so their careers last as long as possible. Your body may not suffer from similar strains and stresses but it will probably benefit from these techniques as much as the professionals.

A word of warning: you'll find a listing about Nutrition in this section because I recognize its importance but there isn't any information about diet or supplements. That's the only subject really not covered in this book, mainly because there are so many different books already available and so many of these therapies have their own nutritional concepts.

Some of you may be a little apprehensive about embarking on a journey into the unknown but fear not. You are more than capable of taking care of yourself in this life! When faced with challenges like buying a new car or a new refrigerator you've been able to do the research, talk with friends and family and make the right decision for your unique situation. This is going to be a similar experience. You know what your problems and needs are better than anyone else and with a little help you're going to discover the best "deal" for your health.

There is one type of map almost everyone is familiar with because they use it on a regular basis - the mall directory map. You start with the knowledge that what you want is in the mall, learning what's available is the first step and the reason you're reading this book. Once you enter the mall and find the directory map you need to look for the red star that shows "You Are Here" in the mall. This is like finding the source of your health problem, it's where you start your journey to better health. Let's assume you're a woman shopping for a new bathing suit at the mall, do you want to shop in a big department store like J.C. Penney or a small specialty boutique like Just Add Water? Both may have a suit for you but they offer different assortments, prices and styles. The comparison would be shopping a big medical system like Traditional Chinese Medicine or a specialty therapy like EFT for better health. Both may have an answer but each has its own features and benefits.

Odds are you're going to shop both because you want to check out sales and the widest selection of options possible. (You know how hard it is to find the perfect bathing suit, or even a good one.) The mall map shows you how to find them with the most direct path. Once in the stores you're going to find some options that you think may work for you but eventually you're to have to try them on. After all, you're a unique person and finding the right cut, style and color to make you look your best takes work, but you're worth it!

If it's that much work to simply find a good bathing suit, how can we expect it to be any easier to find the right therapy for us to find better health? After all, which is more important for you? Learning what's available, finding our red star or beginning at the source of our health problem, navigating the best path to our destination of choice, whether it's finding the perfect bathing suit or better health we use similar steps with different maps.

How are you going to recognize the therapy that you need, your destination? For some people it feels like the proverbial light bulb goes on above their head, that kind of "Ah Ha!" moment when everything seems to fall into place. For many people the light doesn't go on above our head but instead in their heart. After you read a therapy you're going to feel a light, a glow, a kind of warmth that tells you this is something special. It's a special type of attraction but it works for every one of us, it helps lead us to what we need. I know it sounds funny to say you'll recognize it when you see it, but that's what happens. Once it's happened to you, you'll better understand and appreciate how it works. Looking back on my path to better health I can very clearly see the steps I've found along the way that have helped me "unbreak" my health with complementary and alternative therapies.

I wonder how soon you'll discover a therapy to help you improve your health, how quickly you find your path to new hope. To help you along the way there are tips listed and the information in this category is divided into two basic sections: techniques/processes and devices.

TIP

To solve a puzzle/ it's always wise/to find a corner piece/ of any size. /The first one is easy/it's one we all know/eat well for good health/the results always show./ Start with more vegetables/ and more fresh fruits/on these we agree/they are your best routes. /Add more fish/subtract red meat/ down your path to health/you'll be quite fleet.

BODY PROCESSES

ADVANCED ALLERGY THERAPEUTICS

AAT is a non-invasive way to treat seasonal and food allergies along with other health problems. Traditional Chinese Medicine (TCM) allows for the stimulation of specific points on the body which directly accesses each organ system to improve health. These treatment points are located along the spine and correspond with the location of the Sympathetic chain which deals with "fight or flight" responses. By treating reactive organ systems via these points in relation to an offending substance, a reactive state may be treated.

The AAT method does not use needles, but instead utilizes a precision-based acupressure technique for treatment. This unique approach of addressing defensive physiology is highly effective in altering the state of the organ systems. The AAT therapy has been developed as an Integrative Medicine and is utilized by licensed health care professionals who may combine other modalities. However AAT does not claim to cure allergies, nor does the therapy treat the immune system. AAT says that it is a highly effective treatment that provides long-term relief from symptoms associated with allergies or sensitivities.

http://www.allergytx.com/home.html

ADVANCED JAFFE-MELLOR TECHNIQUE™ (JMT)

JMT™ is the abbreviation for Jaffe-Mellor Technique, developed by founders Carolyn Jaffe, Doctor of Acupuncture and Ph.D. candidate in Naturopathy, and Judith Mellor, RN, Ph.D. candidate in Nutrition and certified Chinese medical herbalist. Their combined experience includes various types of acupuncture, herbology and a variety of healing processes.

JMT™ is a bioenergetic therapy that uses **muscle resistance testing** (MRT), a form of applied kinesiology, as the diagnostic tool to identify the pathogenic microorganisms they believe are the cause of many autoimmune diseases. The process may be beneficial for conditions such as osteoarthritis, rheumatoid arthritis, lupus, fibromyalgia, chronic fatigue syndrome, interstitial cystitis, Crohn's disease, colitis, Lyme disease, scleroderma and Multiple Sclerosis. The technique created by Jaffe and Mellor is unique in the way it employs blind testing and focused specific questions to the patient. The original process used vials of materials in the testing process but the process has evolved to the point that vials are no longer used, hence the new designation "advanced".

During the examination, the practitioner views changes in the strength of an isolated muscle against an established baseline. Arm muscles are normally used but any muscle can be used. MRT is valuable as a diagnostic tool because it functions on a subconscious level where the autonomic nervous system resides, the system controlling all bodily functions. In other words, the process looks around behind the conscious mind to see what's happening inside.

Treatment is a gentle tapping of back muscles with either an activator (a chiropractic adjusting instrument) or an arthrostim, a device that provides mild percussion in rapid succession. The technique elicits the proper sensory input to produce more control of body function by the nervous system. The JMT™ protocol allows for as many as ten corrections during any one visit, but the actual number of corrections varies by condition. Practitioners may dispense homeopathic remedies on a temporary basis to help the body eliminate toxic materials that have built up in the tissues as a result of the disease process.

`www.jmttechnique.com`

USER COMMENTS:

♦ In the summer of 2001...I had nine JMT treatments on my very painful right knee...today I have no pain in the knee and I am able to walk up and down stairs easily and do my favorite work in the garden.

♦ I hope many more patients can experience the wonderful relief that JMT offers. Thank you for not only developing this method but also for being willing to train others in the technique.

♦ Five years ago at the age of 21, I suffered from horrible neck/ back pain, migraines, sinus problems, fatigue and joint and muscle stiffness. I felt like my body was decades older than my actual age... During my first treatment, I had mixed feelings because the treatment seemed so very simple. I had to remind myself that the answer is not always a long, drawn out and complex process.

♦ As the practitioner started to diagnose and name the items I was allergic to, I became more and more convinced that this was for real. The items were completely in line with what my blood test had shown. I also had many environmental and chemical allergies of which I was previously unaware. I was starting to get excited and rightfully so. During the next few treatments, I saw some wonderful things.

♦ All of my improvements have maintained for months and I am positive that they are permanent. I look forward with great anticipation to what I will experience as my last few allergies are eliminated. I love telling people about JMT at any opportunity and how it has restored my peace of mind, improved my way of life and given me the freedom to make it whatever I want.

ALEXANDER TECHNIQUE (AT)

Frederick Matthias Alexander (or F.M. Alexander) developed the **Alexander Technique** to help the body to function more efficiently due to his own medical problems. As an actor who developed chronic laryngitis resulting from his performances he was determined to find a way to heal himself. Eventually he discovered that his problem resulted from excess muscle tension and he realized that if neck tension is reduced then the head no longer presses down on the spine so it is free to lengthen.

The process of how we acquire new movements, constantly adapting and changing from our basic, primary motion can cause health problems. As we grow and continually apply these changes we grow numb to how they differ from our natural motions. Alexander called this principle the Debauchery of the Senses but scientists today label it sensory adaptation. The relationship between the neck and head was the Primary Control and the focal point of his work.

The Alexander Technique applies this principle to improve the freedom of movement for the entire body by re-education in new ways to sit, lie down, stand up and other daily functions. By teaching the proper amount of energy for an activity the body retains more energy while maintaining greater balance and coordination. The technique is about unlearning the tension the body has accumulated throughout its lifetime and the resulting muscle tension that produces abnormal mannerisms and motions.

The technique is often taught to improve performance in the arts such as music, acting, dance and even in some sports training. The Julliard School of Performing Arts, the Royal College of Music and the Royal College of Dramatic Art in London are just a few of the institutions teaching this technique. It's also used as therapy to aid the recovery of balance and motion, and for speech training to repair the voice. It's even been used to unlearn repetitive stress and to aid those patients dealing with reduced mobility such as those with Parkinson's disease. Today many professional athletes are beginning to learn this technique because they also want to maximize performance with minimum wear and tear on their body. People of all ages have used the Alexander Technique to improve the quality of their lives for over a century. Training in this self-healing technique is done both by group and individual lessons.

According to the 2007 federal survey 134 responded that they'd used the Alexander Technique in the previous 12 months for a response rate of 0.1%.

Teachers certified by professional societies are often required to complete a 3-year program consisting of more than 1,500 hours of training. Some teachers are trained by an informal, apprentice process. Membership in professional organizations is a matter of personal choice so it is best to learn about any potential Alexander Technique teacher's training prior to beginning any therapy.

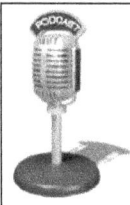

> Robert Rickover has been an Alexander Technique trainer for nearly 30 years and the author of *Fitness Without Stress: A Guide To The Alexander Technique*. You'll hear about a major U.K. study on low back pain showing the Alexander Technique is the most effective therapy over chiropractic therapy and the standard treatment regime of prescription drugs and massage therapy.

www.AlexanderTechnique.com

♦   **USER COMMENTS:** (*by permission from website*)

  ♦ The Alexander Technique helped a long-standing back problem and to get a good night's sleep after many years of tossing and turning.
            —Paul Newman, actor

  ♦ Alexander established not only the beginnings of a far reaching science of the apparently involuntary movements we call reflexes, but a technique of correction and self-control which forms a substantial addition to our very slender resources in personal education.
            —George Bernard Shaw, playwright.

  ♦ I find the Alexander Technique very helpful in my work. Things happen without you trying. They get to be light and relaxed. You must get an Alexander teacher to show it to you.
            —John Cleese, comedian and actor.

  ♦ Mr. Alexander's method lays hold of the individual as a whole, as a self-vitalizing agent. He reconditions and re-educates the reflex mechanisms and brings their habits into normal relation with the functioning of the organism as a whole. I regard this method as thoroughly scientific and educationally sound.
            —Dr. George E. Coghill, Nobel Prize winning anatomist / physiologist.

ANTHROPOSOPHICALLY EXTENDED MEDICINE (AEM)

Anthroposophically Extended Medicine was developed by Rudolf Steiner and Ita Wegman, M.D. in the early 1920s as a holistic approach to medicine. The name describes the fact that all practitioners must first be licensed medical doctors before taking additional training in therapy, alchemy and the spiritual scientific studies outlined by Rudolf Steiner. While it recognizes the accomplishments of Western medicine, it goes further by adding knowledge in the areas of the psyche and spiritual. The synergy from this combination provides for an integrated view of the human being as a living organism.

There are four integrated parts in each human being. First is the Physical Body which is the focus of Western medicine. The second part is called the Etheric Body, which is the higher power that directs the body's growth and regeneration. The third part is the Astral Body, which is what gives us our instincts and the qualities of our soul. The fourth is the unique human concept of Ego, which gives us the power to shape our own destiny. Together they form a framework for diagnosis and therapy.

The major principles of AEM include that Spirit manifests both within human beings and outside in the substances of nature. That wisdom which created nature also works in people. Every substance or process in nature corresponds directly to the inner workings of man.

Art is an indispensable part of life and artistic therapies can strongly affect the disease processes. Every AEM treatment aims to enhance the life force of the patient. This personal power is the basis for improved health along with deepened self-knowledge.

Mistletoe is an example of the use of natural plants and substances. It has been used as a medicine for cancer patients in Europe since 1917. Patients widely use the prescription product in many countries including Germany. The substance is said to support the immune system and improve the quality of life of cancer patients.

The Anthroposophical Spiritual Science is a fundamental part of this approach. Centuries of this knowledge have been developed by monastics, alchemists, Rosicrucians, Auroleus Phillipus Theostratus Bombastus von Hohenheim (known as "Paracelsus") and Christian Friedrich Samuel Hahnemann (the founder of homeopathic medicine) among others. Out of Anthroposophical Medicine, specialized disciplines of Therapeutic Eurythmy, Rhythmical Massage, clay modeling, painting and music therapy have evolved.

In the U.S., the Physicians' Association for Anthroposophical Medicine was founded in 1981. AEM is a leader in the holistic health movement in Europe. *(Also see listing for Therapeutic Eurythmy.)*

`www.paam.net,` `anthroposophy.org`

APPLIED KINESIOLOGY (AK)

Applied Kinesiology (AK) is a technique using muscle testing as a diagnostic tool and for stimulating the body's natural healing ability. Today, there are an estimated 130 variations on this fundamental concept with new adaptations being developed by practitioners frequently. This process is not the same as Kinesiology which is the study of movement or physical activity, although many people have confused the terms.

AK was 'weird' the first time my chiropractor used it on me. The muscle is weak then it's strong, it's just plain strange. Fun but strange!

-Karen

In simple terms, AK uses muscle testing all over the body with no verbal questions and focuses on the structural and nutritional aspects of the body. It also uses gait analysis, range of motion evaluation and other techniques. Many chiropractors, naturopaths, medical doctors, dentists, massage therapists and acupuncturists use the process. Unfortunately the therapy is also used by others interested only in selling supplements and some less-than-reputable healing therapies. Most of the energy or specialized forms of AK use muscle testing as a biofeedback process with only straight-arm (deltoid) muscle tests while asking "yes/no" questions. These practitioners are more concerned about the mental/emotional aspects of the individual.

Although muscle testing had been recognized as far back as the 1920s in the U.S., it wasn't until Dr. George Goodheart made his presentation to an American Chiropractic Association meeting in Denver in 1964 that the term "applied kinesiology" became established. His original observation was that a weak muscle could be treated and the strength immediately improved. At first, his work focused on using muscle testing to improve chiropractic adjustments, but sometimes these treatments were not completely successful so he expanded the diagnostic and treatment options.

He noticed specific relationships between muscles and the energy meridians of Chinese medicine. Weak muscle testing would become strong when a patient touched that part of the body where the dysfunction originated, a process he called therapy localization. The process began to use the body's energy system for rapid healing. From these basic concepts, Applied Kinesiology has grown into a broad field of alternative healing. *Time* magazine named him an Alternative Medicine Innovator for his work.

One of the early pioneers in the field was John F. Thie, a chiropractor in Southern California. When he suggested to Dr. Goodheart in 1965 that his work be made available to the general public, Goodheart told Thie that he should go ahead and do it. Dr. Thie then created **Touch For Health™** (TFH) Kinesiology, publishing *Touch For Health* in 1973 as a self-care approach. Dr. Thie felt the system was so safe and simple that no one needed any training or certification. Today it is one of the most popular types of AK in the world.

TFH muscle testing is a cooperative event involving the practitioner with the active participation by the client or as self-testing. It can be done standing, sitting or lying down and is always done fully clothed. The therapist or person pulls or pushes against a muscle with about two pounds, or light pressure, for two seconds with a limited range of motion of just two inches or less. If the muscle is weak, "squishy" or simply doesn't lock into place, then the energy within the related meridian is probably not in balance. The therapist can then massage the corresponding points on the body to restore normal energy flow and muscle strength. There are five types of energy systems addressed with the TFH process, but practitioners can usually check and balance muscles for all 28 meridians (from Traditional Chinese Medicine) in about 20 minutes. For self-practitioners a daily tune-up using 14 muscles on each side of the body can be done in just a few minutes. Today there is also a computer program to guide TFH treatment.

The International College of Applied Kinesiology (ICAK) was founded in the 1970s and it offers training and certification by its board. Other types of applied kinesiology normally offer their own training and certification programs.

There are many different types of applied kinesiology and this is just a sample. Because different variations use different concepts this subject is categorized for Body, Mind and Energy.

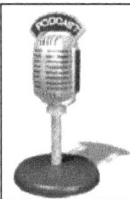

> The Touch For Health system was developed by Dr. John F. Thie and made available to the public in his 1973 book. My interview with his son Matthew Thie, spokesman and advanced Touch For Health instructor, explains more about the technique and its health benefits.

www.tfhka.org

USER COMMENTS:

♦ I have been suffering from osteoarthritis for a number of years in both knees and my left hip. All the doctor could give me to ease the constant pain was Panadeine Forte which I found to be detrimental to my driving capabilities. I was given 15 minutes of Kinergy treatment and I felt the pain leave my body and have had no pain ever since. I also received treatment for my right ankle which used to swell up since being a prisoner of war in 1945. Now there is no sign of the swelling.

♦ During a Kinergetics group my system for hair, skin and nails came up as needing work and was dealt with along with other systems. In the following weeks I noticed changes in an indented scar under my eye [it was 40 years old - acquired from a huge boil I got while an underfed student in the 60s]. Within 3 weeks the scar raised up became sore and then completely disappeared. This was an impressive bonus while working on another issue.

♦ About seven months ago I started sleep-walking, my wife said I should see her kinesiologist since after seeing him she is migraine free after 16 years, so I thought I would give it a try. After the session I told Brett that I had approached four doctors to have them amputate my right leg which was badly damaged in a motorcycle accident 20 years ago. The doctors would not amputate but could not help with the pain. Brett said while I was there would I like to try some Kinergetics pain release on it. I lay back on his table and 15 minutes later I stood up again, the pain had gone from a seven out of ten to a two out of ten. Amazing! I no longer want my leg cut off and I walk four times the distance I could before. Now there is only slight discomfort when I do too much, but is relieved quickly when I rest. It's good to wake up every morning pain free. As for the sleep-walking, I had three session seven months ago and still no sleep-walking. I am amazed that I am pain free after such a long time.

Energy Kinesiology is a term coined by Donna Eden in the 1970s to describe a process of using muscle testing for detecting and correcting imbalances in the body related to stress, nutrition, injuries and even nutritional deficiencies. The Energy Kinesiology Association offers training and certification in its specialty.

`www.energyk.org`

USER COMMENTS:

♦ I told my kinesiologist 'It's just this little issue.' However it took quite a while and another session in the morning but I woke up that Friday (yesterday) and if I stood upright and relaxed my torso would twist. If I really let it relax it would pull my shoulder toward my hip...yes, down. It was amazing to watch. She worked on me with everything she knows and I could track the session by how much twist or discomfort was still there. Inch by inch and pain by pain it all just melted away. Also, on the drive home I got out of the car to go to the rest area and normally I would be stiff from the drive. But I wasn't stiff at all and even more my walk was 'loose'. Meaning that I felt my hips able to have free motion which I don't think I've had since...I don't know when but I think since about 12 years old when the issue/injury we were working on was started. Because I remember in Junior High thinking I developed my "walk" like other girls do at about that age, but later I realized it was from a dance injury that caused tension in my low back so I would throw one hip forward...I just thought it was the way I walked.

Health Kinesiology was created by Jimmie Scott as a brand of bioenergetic kinesiology. The process uses muscle testing to identify the priority of the needed work and which energy balancing methods to use. It also identifies the stresses disrupting the energy flow in the individual. For one of his techniques, the Allergy Tap™, he places a substance over a specific acupuncture point on the belly and taps eight pairs of acupuncture points to identify and cure the allergy. For more information please see

`www.subtlenergy.com`

USER COMMENTS:

♦ My impression is one of enlightenment. I feel that I have started on the next stage in the journey of my life and have left the baggage of my past behind. It has left me with a thirst for more knowledge about HK.

I was impressed by the effectiveness of the techniques, their simplicity and the rapidity in getting results. I am particularly interested in the psychological aspect of HK treatment, as it seems to deal straight to the core of the problem however far in the past or subconscious that may be. The results I have seen so far really motivate me into practicing and make me eager to go on further in the study of HK.

Dawson Program, also known as vibrational kinesiology, was developed by Cameron Dawson. It's based on the concept that the body's emotional, structural, physical and chemical processes are all interrelated so that any change will result in an alteration of the body's energy system. The body contains innate intelligence for constant self-healing and pain and illness are simply a warning system that outside attention is necessary. This process uses muscle testing to locate problems and then applies sound as healing energy.

www.dawsonprogram.com

Neuro Emotional Technique® (NET) was developed by Scott Walker, D.C. and is based on the concept that memories are stored in the body which can negatively affect health. NET practitioners use muscle testing to locate a problem event and then perform chiropractic adjustments, use supplements or homeopathic remedies while the client focuses on the problem.

www.netmindbody.com

USER COMMENTS:

♦ I was amazed that a pain in my shoulder could possibly relate to a hassle with a friend in the 3rd grade and have the pain resolve after NET. That was 15 years ago. Since that time I have been certified in NET and am still amazed how accurate it is and how it shortens my treatment with PTSD clients.

♦ I developed an extreme posture lean to accommodate my acute back pain. I received an NET treatment and not only did the pain disappear but I immediately stood erect and was able to move about effortlessly.

AROMATHERAPY

Aromatherapy is the ancient concept of using potent distilled extracts of flowers, fruits, grasses, leaves, spices, roots, woods and other organic substances to stimulate the organs, the healing systems of the body and to enhance psychological well being. As a holistic healing process it is able to work on several different levels. Using essential oils the approach delivers various scents to the body directly through the skin by massage or inhaled through the nose.

"Women know the importance of smell so this therapy makes sense to me."
- Karen

The use of the olfactory sense provides for an immediate response and easy absorption into the bloodstream, even when the subject has a stuffy nose and can't smell. This pathway is especially powerful because it is the only place in the body where the central nervous system is directly exposed to contact with the environment. Once an olfactory cell is activated it sends a signal directly to the limbic part of the brain. In most cases our subconscious mind has already received and reacted to the signal due to our memories and emotions before we're consciously aware of the sensation.

Essential oils have been used for thousands of years. The Chinese may have been the first to use them along with incense to create harmony and balance. The Egyptians used different types of oils to prepare their dead for entombment, in cosmetics, as medicines and for spiritual purposes. It wasn't until the 16th century that essential oils became available in an apothecary. In 1928, French chemist René-Maurice Gattefossé created the term aromatherapy as part of his work with essential oils. Today, aromatherapy is growing in popularity as part of the return to more natural types of healing. A few drops of essential oils can simply be put on a tissue and inhaled or a professional atomizer may be used. Drops can also be placed on acupuncture points to boost healing or they can be used in massage. Many people are familiar with aromatherapy, they've used Vicks Vaporub, a product that uses eucalyptus.

Essential oils are produced by different techniques depending on the organic source including cold-pressed, steam and the absolute distillation process. Hospitals and nursing homes in America are beginning to use Aromatherapy but clinical studies in the United Kingdom are speeding acceptance in Europe. Properly stored essential oils may last up to 7 years.

The olfactory sense was the subject of the 2004 Nobel Laureate in Physiology or Medicine recognizing that 3% of our genes create olfactory receptor cells which enable human beings to detect 10,000 different odors.

Perfume oils or fragrances are not the same as essential oils since they contain manmade chemicals although there are some natural perfumers. Be aware that synthetic products are available

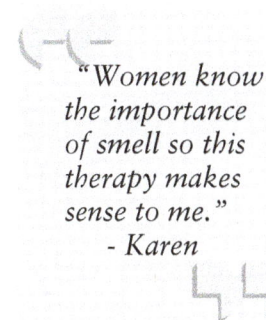

which claim to have aromatherapy properties. As with all products, holistic or not, Buyer Beware is a wise precaution.

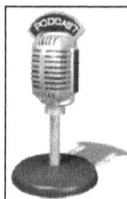

> Listen to Kelly Holland Azzaro, Vice President of the National Association for Holistic Aromatherapy (NAHA), talk about this ancient therapy. She is also a Registered Aromatherapist, a Certified Clinical Aromatherapy Practitioner, a Certified Bach Flower Practitioner and a Licensed Massage Therapist so she has an extensive understanding of this field from everyday experiences to therapeutic applications.

www.naha.org

USER COMMENTS:

♦ Essential oils are always fun to use because they just smell so nice. They can make you feel better physically as well as emotionally. I haven't tried that many of the different scents but it's amazing how each one produces a different and unique reaction.

♦ One of the more interesting uses of essential oils is for energy balancing. For example, they can help restore the power of a chakra. Using a pendulum and specific stones to measure the strength of each chakra you can inhale selected essential oils and immediately retest a weak chakra. You'll find it's suddenly strong and vital again as a result of the essential oil.

♦ Aromatherapy isn't just for the holistic crowd anymore. Today even real estate agents are taught to put a pan of water with vanilla on the stove in a model home to stimulate feelings of warmth and a sense of home. Grocery stores make sure the smell of fresh bread or cakes fill the store. Restaurants want to have the aroma of their best dishes filling the air.

ASIAN BODYWORK THERAPY (ABT)

Asian Bodywork Therapy (ABT) is based upon Traditional Chinese Medicine although some forms only have roots in TCM. Treatments of the body, spirit and mind with ABT involve restoring the flow and balance of the life force or chi (chee) by manipulation and pressure.

The foundation forms of ABT are *Amma*, *Shiatsu* and *Medical Qigong* but today there are many different forms including: *Acupressure*; *AMMA Therapy*®; *Chi Nei Tsang*; *Five Element Shiatsu*; *Integrative Eclectic Shiatsu*; *Japanese Shiatsu*; *Jin Shin Do*® *Bodymind Acupressure*; *Macrobiotic Shiatsu*; *Shiatsu Anma Therapy*; *Nuad Bo Rarn*; *Tuina* and *Zen Shiatsu*.

Acupressure – read the Energy/Spirit book.

Amma – the traditional Korean style of bodywork based upon the Chinese form "Anma". The name means "push-pull" for the style of deep-tissue manipulation used along with acupressure and other points.

Chi Nei Tsang – begins the energy flow in the navel area and then guides the healing power to other parts of the body.

Five Element Shiatsu – relies on the traditional four cornerstones of diagnosis in TCM which are observation, listening, asking and touch. The radial pulse is a key facet of the diagnosis since it often provides crucial information. Locating the disharmony in the body is the basis for determining the best course of treatment.

Integrative Eclectic Shiatsu – combines Japanese Shiatsu with TCM and a Westernized style of soft-tissue manipulation along with dietary and herbal treatments.

Japanese Shiatsu – meaning finger pressure, usually the thumbs, along complete meridian lines.

Jin Shin Do® **Bodymind Acupressure** – uses deep pressure with techniques to focus the mind and body.

Macrobiotic Shiatsu – is based on the belief that every person is a part of nature. Treatment uses hand and bare foot pressure to improve the flow of chi along with dietary guides, medicinal plants, breathing techniques and corrective exercises.

Shiatsu Anma Therapy – combines the energy system of TCM with modern pressure therapy.

Nuad Bo Rarn – is the traditional Thai bodywork style based upon Indian Buddhist medicine and TCM along with a spiritual focus.

Tuina – is a type of Chinese bodywork using soft-tissue massage along with herbal medicines and therapeutic exercises.

Zen Shiatsu – The American Organization for Bodywork Therapies of AsiaTM (AOBTA®) is the main professional organization for this field, but the National Certification Commission for Acupuncture and Oriental Medicine (NCCAOM) provides the entry certification for ABT. **www.aobta.org**

USER COMMENTS:

♦ I was introduced to shiatsu by a friend who was training to become a practitioner. Lucky me! She used me for practice. I had had some "ordinary" massage before, but shiatsu immediately felt special. My learner-friend was methodical and went down the "points" on either side of the spine, and I started feeling my body in new ways. I loved it.

But that was the end of it until I came to Louisiana and came down with cancer. After my recovery I decided I needed to take better care of myself, and I remembered shiatsu. No two sessions are ever the same with my new practitioner. She takes an inventory beforehand and then magically addresses whatever is ailing me at the time. Magical is a good word for what happens: with astonishingly little pressure, she manages to effect profound changes. I always follow the process with amazement and gratitude, as on a journey, new each time, of discovery of my own body.

I'm convinced, since my cancer these twice-monthly sessions have kept me healthy. If I miss a session I begin to feel it fairly soon. With my intense high-pressure job I crave the release and nurturing of the shiatsu touch and process. It gives me energy and balance and peace. It gives me joy! After every session I wish everyone could have such an experience. The world would be a better, more peaceful place!

AUDITORY INTERVENTION TECHNIQUE (AIT)

Dr. Guy Bérard developed an auditory stimulation technique in the 1960s in France following his work with Dr. Alfred Tomatis and the Audio-Psycho-Phonology approach (or **Tomatis Method**). Practitioners introduced the **Bérard Method of Auditory Intervention Training** to the U.S. in 1991 as a method to help people with learning disabilities, autism, ADD and other conditions. Dr. Bérard's book, *Hearing Equals Behavior*, was translated into English in 1992.

"I really hate taking drugs. There are so many risks, I prefer to find a more natural way."
- Karen

The premise is that certain people hear differently which impacts their ability to learn and their behavior including motor functions. Dr. Bérard felt that ear function needs to be balanced just like eyes and hands. By using filters to decrease the volume of those frequencies which a person hears too acutely (or peaks) and then randomly modulating frequencies during listening sessions, the AIT sound amplifier can retrain the brain's hearing process. Today the minimum age for this process is 3 years old.

Practitioners normally take audiograms before, at the mid-point, and at the completion of the sessions to identify and adjust the problem frequencies. The listener will experience 18 to 20 listening sessions of 30 minutes each over a 10- to 20-day period. It's common for people to double up the sessions and have two sessions per day for 10 days. During the listening sessions, the person listens to specially processed music tuned for their hearing situation.

Scientists have found that filtering peaks for the developmentally disabled population is optional since it is the modulation, not the filtering, that is critical for them. The best results normally involve using a multi-disciplinary approach which could include specialists in the fields of audiology, psychology, special education, and speech/language. There are other types of auditory intervention training programs that use different types of equipment.

Another type of AIT is the **Samonas Method**. Developed by German sound engineer Ingo Steinbach, it combined the ideas of Tomatis with advances in both technology and physics.

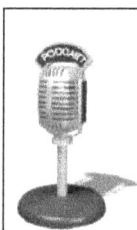

> Sally Brockett is the President of the Berard Auditory Intervention Training International Society, Director of the IDEA Training Center and a Berard AIT Instructor and Practitioner for 17 years. Sally was trained by Dr. Guy Berard, the creator of the technique, and upon his retirement he appointed her his world-wide representative with responsibility for his program. Parents with children who have ADD, autism or other problems will want to hear this one ... so will adults with ADD.

`www.BerardAITwebsite.com`

USER COMMENTS:

♦ From a parent about her child): He has changed so much, more than any other year! He gained in social skills, emotional, speech, transitions…His speech therapist has been with him for three years and has never seen him improve as much as he did since AIT. She is truly amazed. He could not write his name before, but within two weeks after AIT he was writing his name. At school he sits in Circle Time; every year before this year he could not sit in Circle Time or any group activity because he said the kids hurt his ears. Now he enjoys all group activities. Now he talks about his friends and he has them over. He used to hate kids touching him, now he just loves his friends. It has been a remarkable year, one of incredible gains for him. Now he is finally ready for kindergarten! Thank you for opening a wonderful new world for our son.

♦ I continue to be amazed at the differences AIT has made in my life. I came for AIT in the hope of improving my ability to learn a foreign language. I am pleased to say that everything I had hoped for concerning my ability to learn another language was achieved. My auditory memory/learning ability has also increased. Not only can I repeat longer phrases in French, but I can remember a phone number when someone says it! Also, my vocabulary is less 'visually dependent'. In a conversation I now 'hear what you mean' instead of only 'seeing what you mean'.

♦ Also, I am remarkably more comfortable with other people. To the observer there was nothing in my behavior that would have revealed my discomfort. Indeed, others, especially in business, described me as "an extrovert", someone who was remarkably at ease with others. Not the case. Within, I always felt "different" than others. I knew that I preferred to be by myself. Social events that were fun for others were not particularly fun for me. After a few hours of socializing, I was more than ready to be by myself. Before AIT I had never realized how extremely uncomfortable I had been. After AIT, I came to realize that social exchanges formerly left me vibrating. I only recognized this when the vibrating stopped! I think that I was in a constant "system overload", which I only recognized once it was gone.

♦ I wish Bérard AIT had been available to me as a child. It would have saved me from a lot of heartache.

AUTOGENICS TRAINING (AT)

Autogenics Training (AT) is a self-help technique to generate physical relaxation, bodily health and mental peace. German physician Johannes Schultz first published the approach in 1932. The term means "self regulation" because it deals with controlling breathing, heart rate, blood pressure and other body functions. It can also be beneficial in overcoming addictions such as smoking as well as to change behaviors and to resolve anxieties.

It can take people up to three months to learn and become proficient with the process. Generally, the training sequence involves a progression of steps at regular intervals. You can learn and become proficient in the Warm Up phase in just a few days. However, the first two sequences, often called Heaviness and Warmth, may require three weeks of practice each. The next four steps (Calm Heart, Breathing, Stomach and Cool Forehead) each require two weeks of practice.

While Shultz compared the technique to yoga and meditation, it deals with the body without any mysticism. It is a method of training the body's autonomic nervous system. Experts believe it functions in a similar manner to biofeedback, the relaxation response or self-hypnosis.

Autogenics is said to be far more effective than simple Progressive Muscle Relaxation (PMR) so it's worth the investment of time and effort to learn the technique. You can also modify the process to deal with specific issues and problems by inserting visualizations of the negative behavior, its detrimental effects on your life and then a positive visualization of your life without the behavior. For maximum effectiveness, it should be practiced on a daily basis.

`www.autogenic-therapy.org.uk`

AYURVEDA

Ayurveda in Sanskrit means "The Science of Life" and it's believed to be more than 5,000 years old making it one of the oldest health systems in the world. Developed in India, Ayurvedic medicine focuses on developing a balance of mind, body and spirit to maintain health and prevent illness. Each person is unique, with an individual energy signature, their own mix of physical, mental and emotional characteristics. Proper thinking, lifestyle, diet and herbs are used to achieve proper balance for each person. There are many similarities between Ayurveda and Traditional Chinese Medicine (TCM).

The vital energy of a person is called **Prana** which is centered around the energy centers in the body called **Chakras**. Unlike the Chinese system of Yin/Yang, the Indian energy system has three separate elements or doshas:

- **Vata Dosha** – composed of space and air, it is the energy of movement.
- **Patta Dosha** – is made of fire and water, it's the body's metabolic processes.
- **Kapha Dosha** – is the glue that holds it together, the body's structure represented by earth and water.

Ayurveda uses a holistic approach with therapies that appeal to all of the senses to treat each individual. Practitioners may use Taste (herbs and nutrition); Touch (massage, yoga, exercise); Smell (aromatherapy); Sight (color therapy); Hearing (music therapy, mantra meditation, chanting) and Spiritual therapy. The system is about more than just health, it's about living.

In many cases, a practitioner will begin by recommending a **Panchakarma** or cleansing process to eliminate the accumulated toxins in the body. **Basti** refers to giving medications rectally to treat **vata dosha**, or problems related to Vata by cleansing the colon. **Nasya** means giving medications nasally and may be either wet or dry. **Virechana** means cleansing of the pitta through the lower pathways.

In the U.S. today, Ayurveda positions itself as a complement to Western medicine, a way to prevent illness by reducing stress and maintaining balance so the body's own defenses can function effectively. According to the 2007 government survey the number of people utilizing Ayurveda in the previous 12 months has increased from the 2002 survey but still remains about 0.1% of the population.

`http://www.ayurvedanama.org/`

USER COMMENTS:

- ♦ This healing system is completely individualized and comprehensive. It's about what type of body you have and the healthiest lifestyle for you. Imbalance in the body leads to disease and malfunction so everything is about maintaining balance. Since I'm a "patta" or fire, I have to cut down on spicy foods in the summer. Ayurveda isn't interested in putting a particular name on a disease, they want to know the cause of the problem. They realize that the same set of symptoms can come from a variety of imbalances depending on each individual, which is why they're so focused on each person. They'll check your tongue, fingernails, all sorts of tests and talk with you about your life and lifestyle to completely learn who you are before trying to determine what the source of the problem really is. Individual differences also make a huge difference in their prescriptions to improve your health depending on your body.

♦ This process focuses on the body's normal functions which are so often stymied in America. We have air conditioning so we don't sweat toxins from our body. We go to the bathroom on breaks, not when we want to, frustrating the body's attempt to eliminate waste and toxins in a timely manner which leads to plaque buildup in the colon. You can see how it's not hard to let toxins build up to the point that there is a problem.

♦ There is even balance for the mind and spirit as well since too much media can cause imbalance in that part of your total body system. They believe in a media fast to create balance since many diseases (smoking, alcoholism, etc.) can result from mental imbalances. They also use a head massage with oils to cool the head so the body can function properly. Massage, especially with oils, is a big part of their process because it helps them move toxins around and out of the body.

♦ These herbs are an organic part of my 'medicine cabinet' and many have gained respect from other Western scientists.

♦ As a limo driver I never leave my car. I drive and eat in the seat and get no exercise. My stomach was hurting and not digesting any foods. The Fire Harmony has improved my digestion and I get out stretching once in a while.

BEE-VENOM THERAPY (BVT)

Bee-Venom Therapy (BVT), also called bee-sting therapy, is one type of Apitherapy or the therapeutic use of beehive products such as honey or royal jelly. The use of bees and bee products goes back to ancient Egypt, Greece and China but Hungarian doctor Bodog Beck popularized the treatment in the 1930s.

It's believed that bee stings work to stimulate the body's immune system in specific locations, training it to become stronger each time, a process similar to a weight lifter increasing weights at each workout. It may also increase the body's production of cortisol. Bee stings are commonly thought to ease the symptoms of arthritis, MS, fibromyalgia, irritable bowel syndrome (IBS) and other conditions.

BVT may use up to 80 stings per day with live bees by urging them to sting the affected area, on trigger points or acupuncture centers. The therapy normally is used about three times per week with a gradual increase in the number of stings. The highest potency bee venom comes directly from a live bee in the late spring or early fall. Standardized bee venom solution may also be injected or can be used in a cream or ointment. Bee venom is a complex source of peptides, enzymes with at least 18 active components which have pharmaceutical properties although the exact mechanism of its function is unknown. It's also a volatile substance which may lose potency from a variety of factors.

Because about 2% of the population may have allergic reactions to bee stings the first step is to test the risk factor by injecting a very small amount of bee venom underneath the skin or with a single bee sting. If no allergic reaction develops the therapy continues by testing a little more venom. In any case it is always a smart idea for anyone using BVT to have a bee sting kit with a syringe of epinephrine close at hand for safety. Even if you haven't had a problem with the first 79 stings doesn't mean you won't have a problem with the 80ᵗʰ. Allergic reactions can include anaphylactic shock which can be fatal. Bee venom has been approved by the FDA for desensitization purposes only.

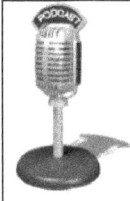

> Frederique Keller is the President of the American Apitherapy Society, a bee keeper for over 20 years, a licensed acupuncturist and a medical herbalist. Our conversation covered a wide range of benefits from our friends the amazing honey bees beginning with Bee Venom Therapy.

www.apitherapy.org, www.beevenom.com

USER COMMENTS:

♦ Who could have predicted my diagnosis of MS in early 2000? At 53, I was healthy and fit and joyous ... I knew immediately that I would never take any drugs, as I was dubious of the illness anyway and felt totally uncomfortable introducing a serious manufactured drug-company product into my energetic living system... (so my beekeeper) began stinging my feet and spine over a period of two years. During these past few years, the story of apitherapy and the bees has been my manifesto. I sing it across backyards and in coffee shops. The journey has been wondrous. I am healthier than ever. I have hope, energy, and curiosity about the future and am ready to spread the word of the healing power of the hive.

TIP

If the Mountains of Misery block your start/ my advice – don't strain your heart/ don't climb over the snowy crest/ an easier path is always best. The answer to the challenge is easy to see/ a canyon-shaped therapy is the key.

BIOACOUSTICS THERAPY

BioAcoustics Therapy is different from other types of sound therapies due to its use of human voice analysis. The concept is that our voices are a representation of our state of health. Voice analysis equipment detects frequencies the person emits, also called a "signature sound", which represents the vibrational energies of the body. Once altered vibrations due to physical or mental illness are detected by voice analysis the body's energy field is then harmonized by listening to the corrected personal sound frequencies.

Sounds have been used for healing since ancient times (see Crystal Bowl Therapy). The use of this particular type of Bioacoustics as a therapeutic technique originated with Sharry Edwards in 1982. The International Association of New Sciences awarded Sharry their top honor – Scientist of the Year - in 2001 for her leadership in the field of BioAcoustics and Sound Health.

http://www.soundhealthoptions.com/

BIOENERGETIC ANALYSIS

Bioenergetic Analysis or simply **Bioenergetics** is a therapy that uses both the body and the mind to help resolve emotional problems and to help people discover the joy in living. The core principle is the body represents the person - what affects the body affects the mind and the mind affects the body. Muscular patterns in the body, movement and even breathing patterns offer diagnostic tools for the bioenergetic psychotherapist who uses this information to develop a framework for the course of therapy. Events in childhood play an especially vital element in the process since they impact adult life and relationships.

From breathing to handshake to types of movement, each motion of the body offers diagnostic and therapeutic opportunities with this process. Body work as part of the therapy program may take several different forms. For example, Therapeutic Touch is used to facilitate the process. Bioenergetics provides increased awareness of the body, the feelings connected to the sensations and to better appreciate how these relate to events in your life.

Dr. Alexander Lowen is the founder of Bioenergetic Analysis. His original work *Bioenergetics* followed his studies with Wilhelm Reich, M.D., an early student of Sigmund Freud, in the early 1940s.

The International Institute for Bioenergetic Analysis was created in 1956 as a membership organization to certify practitioners, provide continuing education and advance the art and science of Bioenergetic Analysis.

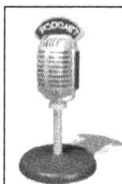

> Rick Spletter is the President of the Dallas Society for Bioenergetic Analysis and also a trainer for the organization. He's been using Bioenergetic Analysis with his clients for 30 years so our conversation featured some interesting anecdotes from his experiences.

`www.bioenergetic-therapy.com`

USER COMMENTS:

- After years of trying many forms of therapy and medication, I attended a lecture about Bioenergetic Analysis. My 'inner child' was drawn to the therapist, and my intellect decided this was a modality worth trying. Bioenergetics allowed me to reach places inside that nothing else had reached. Because much of my abandonment issues originated before I had language, the trauma was stored in my body, and no talk therapy could reach it. After much hard work, I finally began liking myself, felt I deserved to be loved and treated with respect, and sensed contact with a Higher Power who wanted the best for me.

- I have been Rolfed, used Acupuncture, Acupressure, and bioenergetic bodywork which have changed my life. The bioenergetic bodywork deals with both mind and body. I have more energy, think clearly and feel more grounded since I experienced this process. I liked the process so much that I did the training to become a certified bioenergetic therapist.

BIOFEEDBACK

Biofeedback is a process of recognizing the functioning of the body's systems in real time with the goal of correcting or improving performance. Change is accomplished by learning to modify the mind-body connection to alter muscle response, blood pressure and other bodily functions. The concept of voluntarily changing the autonomic nervous system through feedback was first studied in 1961. According to the latest federal study on complementary and alternative medicine the number of Americans reporting they'd used biofeedback in the previous 12 months increased from 0.1% in the 2002 national survey to 0.2% in 2007.

Many people are familiar with the high-tech equipment often used in movies and sports to improve muscle tone and coordination but a mirror can also be a biofeedback device. When a person simply watches the reflection of each step, they're learning to modify the signals from their mind to their body to improve walking. Whether the feedback is done with visual images, sounds or both, it is a process to focus attention to learn improved control.

There are non-invasive devices that will measure muscle tension and brain waves for biofeedback. The term also includes other processes such as:

- **Electromyography (EMG)** – a specialized device used to measure muscle tension, often used as therapy for headaches, morning stiffness and fibromyalgia.

- **Thermal** – the measurement of skin temperature has been found beneficial for Raynaud's Disease and other conditions involving reduced blood flow. It's also used to treat migraines.

- **GSR** – Galvanic Skin Response is a measurement of the skin's conductivity, usually connected with an audible signal that becomes higher when stressed and lower when relaxed.

- **HRV** - Heart Rate Variability measures changes in heartbeat as a biofeedback tool.

- **Respiration Training** – uses various technologies to train and control respiration.

- **Electroencephalography** or **EEG** biofeedback, also known as **Neurofeedback**, which measures brainwaves by sensors attached to the scalp and each ear. Brain frequency activity is presented so specific frequencies can be stimulated or reduced. The technique has been found beneficial for many problems including ADD, learning difficulties, depression and chronic fatigue.

The technique has a wide variety of uses. It's used by coaches to improve sports performance, by specialists to improve urinary incontinence, to help stroke victims regain functionality, to help people learn to relax, and for chronic pain and headaches. It's also the basis for most anger management programs. A popular feature of biofeedback therapy is dealing with stress. However scientists still cannot explain exactly how biofeedback actually works.

The use of the term biofeedback started in the late 1960s but certification by the Biofeedback Certification Institute of America began in 1981. There are many state associations which also list biofeedback professionals.

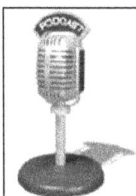

> Listen to a podcast with John G. Arena, Ph.D., President of the Association for Applied PsychoPhysiology and Biofeedback to discover the strategies and uses of this therapy. Dr. Arena is also the Lead Psychologist at the Veterans Hospital in Augusta, Georgia and Professor of Psychiatry and Health Behavior at the Medical College of Georgia.

www.aapb.org

USER COMMENTS:

- My severe tinnitus was making my life miserable. Work was difficult. Reading, thinking, and especially sleeping were a problem. Thanks to Biofeedback therapies I now enjoy life again. Thank you Biofeedback Therapies!

- Our grandson has many health issues including ADHD, bipolar, anger and behavior problems and a brain injury from birth. We were told about Biofeedback Therapies and decided to give it a try. After just a few sessions we noticed a change, he would still get angry but not as long as before. Now he uses the technique he learned when he feels himself getting angry at school or at home and he is able to find the "calm place" that he learned. This has been a miracle for our grandson!

BIORESONANCE THERAPY (BRT)

Bioresonance Therapy (BRT) uses electromagnetic frequencies produced by the body to detect and eliminate health problems. Science knows that all living cells radiate weak electromagnetic energy similar to brain waves. BRT measures this energy to determine healthy and unhealthy conditions along with reactions to specific substances (food, bacteria, and toxins). Practitioners amplify healthy signals and return them to the body to strengthen normal body functions. Unhealthy signals are inverted by a mirror circuit and returned to the body through electronic mats to cancel out the harmful energy. This is the same type of wave cancellation theory used in noise reduction headphones.

The concept for this process is that substances which stress or strain your energetic system are the cause of illness and disease, but it is usually a cumulative effect of several stress factors. Identifying and relieving the major stresses to the system will allow the body to handle the minor ones. Allergy treatments usually take two sessions while infections may take two to four visits. Chronic conditions may require up to eight sessions.

The technology attracted attention in 1991 when Dr. Peter Schumacher used it effectively to neutralize allergies. Study into the concept began in 1923 with the work of Russian scientist Alexander Gurwitsch, but it was German physicist Dr. F.A. Popp who proved the existence of light emission (bio-photons) from living cells in 1975. Franz Morell and Erich Rasche introduced Bioresonance Therapy in 1977 with the launch of the MORA-Therapy device. Today there are thousands of BRT machines of many different designs in use around the world by doctors, dentists and even veterinarians to treat a variety of disorders.

The FDA has banned some of these devices from the US market.

www.bioresonance.uk.com

BONNIE PRUDDEN MYOTHERAPY®

In 1976 Bonnie Prudden developed her **Myotherapy** method to relax muscle spasms, relieve pain and improve circulation. The technique is based on the concepts of trigger point injection therapy and therapeutic exercise. The term comes from "myo" for muscle and "therapy" for treatment.

"Trigger points" can begin in a muscle whenever it is damaged and are activated by either emotional or physical stress causing the muscle to spasm with pain. The basic formula is:

Trigger Points + Stress + Triggering Mechanism = Chronic Pain.

Older people often suffer from trigger points more as a result of collecting more trigger points throughout their lives. Bonnie used to say it's pain that ages us, not years, and pain comes from someplace, usually trigger points. Fibromyalgia is a type of muscle pain that can be helped by this therapy.

Myotherapists defuse the pain by pressing or pinching on the appropriate trigger point for several seconds with fingers, knuckles or even elbows and then passively stretching the muscle into its normal relaxed and painless condition. Usually the pressing lasts less than seven seconds at each spot. Patients wear loose clothing and no shoes for a myotherapy session. The exercises taught to each patient afterwards are necessary for them to remain pain free. Normally patients require less than ten sessions for relief and they'll have the knowledge of how to use the therapy on themselves using tools like the Bodo and the Shepherd's Crook. The technique can even be used on animals.

Bonnie Prudden's Myotherapy® method is taught in person and through her many books, videos and media appearances. Her work on physical fitness began with her research on the nation's school children in the 1950s which she reported to President Dwight Eisenhower. As a result of her efforts the federal government established the first requirements for children's fitness programs. As a result of all of her work she received the President's Council Lifetime Achievement Award in 2007.

Bonnie Prudden Myotherapy is a registered trademark of Bonnie Prudden Myotherapy, Inc.

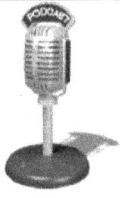

> My conversation with 95-year-old Bonnie Prudden was delightful. It's not often I get to talk with a living legend! She says that pain is what ages us and her therapy can relieve 95% of muscle pain. Listen to Bonnie explain how to use her therapy and what it can do for you. Discover the secret to "Ouch Then Ah" and start moving! She passed away at home in Tucson on December 11, 2011.

www.bonnieprudden.com

USER COMMENTS:

♦ I call it a recipe book on trigger points and recommend the book (Pain Erasure the Bonnie Prudden Way) to all my patients.

♦ I learned that there is always hope and that I am not stuck in my current condition.

♦ I now have reliable information that can easily be incorporated into my work to benefit myself and my clients

BOWEN THERAPY

The Bowen Therapy is a bodywork system that uses cross-fiber muscle movements throughout the body. Tom Bowen created the process in Australia. He was untrained in formal therapy education but had a gift for healing. He began his treatment practice of soft tissue manipulation in the late 1950s and spent his life continually developing his philosophy of healing and his techniques. Unfortunately, he never got around to writing any of it down so today there is some disagreement over his techniques.

The first moves of the Bowen Therapy are done on the back and hips while the client lies face down with only their shoes removed. This initial sequence allows the body to relax, improves the flow of oxygen and circulation while releasing toxins. The series of "moves" in this process are done in a precise sequence across muscle and connective tissues, up and down the body, with the client changing to a face-up position halfway through the treatment. There are short waiting periods during the session which allow the brain to appreciate what's happening and to create a positive response. Sessions usually run 45-60 minutes. The key to the Bowen Therapy is in opening up the body's energy pathways to allow it to heal itself.

Tom Bowen died in 1982 but one of his students, Ossie Rentsch, taught Milton J. Albrecht who was the first Bowen therapist certified outside of Australia. Milton Albrecht sponsored the first Bowen seminar held in the U.S. in 1989. Albrecht founded the Bowen Therapy International organization in 1997 for the competency, certification and quality control of Bowen Therapy practitioners.

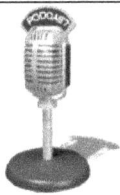

> Tom Bowen developed a unique style of therapy in Australia in the mid-1950s, and today there are several techniques based on his work. I spoke with Deni Larimore Albrecht, administrative director of Bowen Therapy International, about how this technique came to America. She and her late husband Milton sponsored the first Bowen seminar held outside of the South Pacific in 1989.

http://parkerschoolofbowentherapy.com/

USER COMMENTS:

♦ Your Bowen Technique has saved my life! I cancelled my hip surgery scheduled for next week.

♦ I was having some shoulder pain and restriction several years ago when I happened to be having breakfast with a good friend who is also a Bowen Therapist. She offered to do some work on my shoulder right in the parking lot of the restaurant. A few simple moves and the pain and discomfort were gone and have never returned.

♦ Three visits and the amazing Bowen treatment fixed my frozen shoulder. Thanks!

BRAIN BALANCE PROGRAM™

The **Brain Balance Program**™ was developed by Dr. Robert Melillo, neurologist, and author of *Disconnected Kids*. It is designed for children dealing with physical, cognitive or mental, and/or behavioral difficulties or disorders like ADD/ADHD, autism, dyslexia, etc. The therapy is based on the concept that such disorders are the result of imbalances or under-connectivity of the brain as reported in the 2009 study, *Autistic Spectrum Disorders as Functional Disconnection Syndrome* Dr. Robert Melillo and Dr. Gerry Leisman. These problems occur as a result of poor communication between the two hemispheres of the brain or between major neurological networks. Fortunately the brain is capable of growing and changing due to the principle of neuroplasticity.

The program is available only at authorized Brain Balance centers which are learning centers, not health care facilities. The program utilizes a multi-faceted approach to treatment beginning with the assessment of each child's unique situation. In addition to learning skills, testing may include vision, hearing, behavior, diet and other factors. An individualized development program is then designed to meet their needs. The primary focus of the program involves 36 sessions directed towards specific math and reading skills to stimulate specific areas of weakness in the child in order to balance brain performance. Depending on the individual additional 12-week sessions may be required.

www.brainbalancecenters.com

USER COMMENTS:

♦ (My daughter) was not developing the way she should. She didn't crawl properly and every milestone was significantly delayed. The doctors that were treating her felt she had a genetic or chromosome disease, and they gave us no hope that she would be at least normal. Dr. Melillo and his staff at The Brain Balance Center were the only people that listened and addressed her problems… We began sessions and the changes were instantaneous. Tears of joy come when I think about the progress she has made. She began to speak. She moved with more fluidity. She expressed her needs. She was a new little person. This affected my entire family. The doctors who were convinced that she had a genetic disorder (even though all genetic testing was negative or inconclusive) were astonished. They never believed she would be normal, and they had never seen such changes before in a child with her problems.

♦ My son was diagnosed with AD/HD at 6 ½ years old. The Neurologist insisted he be put on medication. We were totally against it. (My son) was very hyperactive, impulsive, and was already having problems focusing and behaving in kindergarten. We are well past half the program and we have seen remarkable changes. He is now calmer, more focused, more cooperative, he listens better, and is less impulsive. His physical body has greatly improved and he feels stronger and more confident. If he does act up at school, the teacher says she corrects him and he stops. Before, he had to be constantly reminded. I recommend this program due to simply…it works.

BRAIN GYM® or Educational Kinesiology (Edu-K)

Brain Gym® was developed over a 25-year period by Paul Dennison, Ph.D. and his wife Gail E. Dennison to help children and adults learn more effectively, especially those diagnosed as learning disabled. Beginning in the 1970s practitioners of the process began to use posture and movement to improve academic, interpersonal and physical learning skills. Today, the process uses 26 specific activities that integrate body and mind to produce quick improvements.

They describe the brain as functioning in three dimensions. "Laterality" means the ability of the brain to coordinate both sides of the brain, a fundamental skill to be able to read, write and communicate. "Focus" concerns the coordination of the brain from front to back, critical for comprehension. "Centering" is about the ability of the brain to coordinate the top and bottom areas. This function is vital for organizational skills and the ability to feel and express emotions. Many of the Brain Gym® activities are based on the relationship of movement to perception and their impact on motor and academic skills.

A private session with a trained Brain Gym® instructor or consultant usually lasts 1-2 hours. Each five-step process or "balance" will remove a block and create a bridge in the brain for that specific learning or action goal. The process promotes the ability to learn at a deep, whole-brained level. Short balances may take only five minutes while a longer balance may take an hour or more.

Brain Gym® is a registered trademark of Brain Gym® International / Educational Kinesiology Foundation.

www.BrainGym.org

USER COMMENTS:

♦ Recently, I started to knit a sweater for my granddaughter. The design was an Aran style with cables, diamonds, and bobbles. I soon found myself having dreadful trouble, and had to undo my stitches again and again. So many fruitless attempts! I was ready to give in; no more fancy knitting for me! Then I said to myself, "This is quite ridiculous. I have knitted incredible patterns for years, and I don't believe that you lose this ability just by getting old." As I sat looking at the pattern for the sweater, I thought, "Hang on just a minute, I need to do some Brain Gym." So I stopped and did 20 minutes of Brain Gym activities. No more trouble! The sweater is now finished and much admired, and I've knitted a couple more for my grandson. What's age got to do with it?

♦ We cannot believe the improvement in our daughter after five sessions. Before we were referred to you our daughter could not tie her shoes without help, could not ride her bike without training wheels, and was having difficulty reading at her grade level. Since working with you she is riding her bike without assistance and training wheels. She is tying her shoes by herself, but most important her reading rate and reading fluency have greatly increased, which has also increased her reading comprehension.

♦ We feel that Brain Gym provided the missing link so she could integrate all the previous therapy. Because of your work, she's made huge improvements academically and socially in a very short time period. We are very grateful for your work and thankful that God sent you into our lives.

BREATHWORK

Breathwork or **conscious breathing** has many different techniques under a variety of names. **Rebirthing**, also called **Rebirthing Breathwork**, is a special breathing technique based on the concept that breathing energy along with air has therapeutic effects on the body. The increase of physical and spiritual energy has a cleansing effect on the body. It is a process to increase awareness of emotions in order to resolve the effects of the past, reconnecting the mind and the body.

Rebirthers don't believe that the past has to be the pattern for the future. It's human nature to suppress those aspects of ourselves that we dislike so we hide feelings of pain, guilt, shame and other negative emotions. Relief is possible using a technique called conscious connected breathing, also known as circular breath, where the client lies on their back or side breathing in and out without a pause. This technique is said to energize the individual with a build up of Chi or life energy. Initially this process is intended for use with a trained and experienced Rebirthing facilitator because this energy could feed negative patterns, which is why Rebirthers provide positive affirmations during the process. Sessions can last one to two hours and many practitioners recommend weekly meetings for at least the first ten sessions.

Many clients do get to re-experience their birth but it isn't the goal of the process. The priority of Rebirthing is to put people in touch with their experience in this moment in time and space, not to offer some type of regression.

Leonard Orr developed Rebirthing in the early 1970s in San Francisco using bathtubs and hot tubs. Eventually the process developed as a dry process to integrate painful experiences from a person's past. He founded Rebirthing Breathwork International, also called Rebirth International, in 1975. Today this organization offers a wide range of training programs.

`www.rebirthingbreathwork.com`

USER COMMENTS:

♦ I tried Rebirthing to try and deal with some emotional issues, hoping to find a way to deal with some very traumatic events in my past, especially my childhood. While breathing isn't hard to do, bringing up horrible experiences and feelings right out of a nightmare can be. I went to the sessions week after week and everything just kept getting worse instead of better. I finally quit and discovered a different process which helped me take the sting out of my experiences and build positive, reinforcing new subconscious beliefs about myself and my life.

Holotropic Breathwork™ was developed by Stanislav Grof, M.D., and Christina Grof in the mid-1970s. Participants breathe deeper and faster than normal for two to three hours, while lying with eyes closed, and listening to evocative music arranged in a specific way. Facilitators, who are certified after extensive training, do not attempt to guide the session; instead participants are encouraged to allow the expression of whatever set of experiences are brought to them by their "inner healers," and facilitators support that expression if needed.

`www.holotropic.com`

CHELATION THERAPY

Chelation Therapy uses di-sodium **EDTA** to remove mercury, lead, cadmium and other toxic metals from the blood by intravenous infusion, pill or other form. The solution may also be combined with other substances such as vitamins. The process is used for treating atherosclerosis and other health problems following testing of blood, urine or hair to diagnose the need for the treatment.

Decades ago scientists thought that hardened arteries might be softened if the calcium in their walls could be removed, which was the basis for initiating the EDTA treatment. The first indication that EDTA might be beneficial for atherosclerosis came in 1956 when the first reports from doctors announced that patients felt better after treatment. The book *Bypassing Bypass* states that six million chelation treatments have been given safely over the last forty years but it includes warnings of serious side effects.

The 2002 federal study on the use of complementary and alternative medicine in America showed that 0.1% had ever used chelation therapy while 0.01% had used it in the previous year. In the 2007 survey use during the prior year increased to 0.02%. The therapy is promoted by the American College for Advancement in Medicine (ACAM).

`www.acam.org, http://www.webmd.com/balance/tc/chelation-therapy-topic-overview`

USER COMMENTS:

♦ EDTA chelation therapy saved my life 2 years ago. I was a hypertensive mess in congestive heart failure taking upwards of 40 Nitroglycerine tablets, as well as high doses of lasix daily just to survive. Since completing therapy I have not used Nitroglycerine in 2 years and only rarely (say 6 months apart) do I use a lasix for excess water retention. This after doctors tried to get me to have Percutaneous Coronary angioplasty with stent placements.

CHIROPRACTIC

The principle of **chiropractic** is that energy, especially of the nervous system, must flow freely through the spinal column for good body health. The relationship of the spine's structure and function to the health of the body is a concept that goes back thousands of years to writings in ancient Greece and China. Even Hippocrates, the Greek physician, (of the Hippocratic Oath for doctors) mentioned the importance of the spine to health.

Chiropractors practice a hands-on technique of healthcare which most people recognize for spinal manipulation or adjustment. The treatment has also been used effectively for a variety of health problems including asthma and IBS. Whether an injury is from a single event such as lifting something heavy or from a repetitive stress of poor posture, the result is physical and chemical changes that restrict the movement of the spine. Manipulation, whether manual or by device, restores mobility which reduces pain, muscle tightness and inflammation so the body can heal. Chiropractors often use what's called "passive muscle testing" meaning they observe the lengthening or shortening of the legs or arms in reaction to touching a specific spot to locate the area needing adjustment.

Chiropractic is the largest, most heavily regulated, and best recognized of CAM professions. There are an estimated 60,000 chiropractors in America today. The therapy was developed by Daniel David Palmer in Davenport, Iowa in 1895. He began the Palmer School of Chiropractic in 1897 and it continues to be one of the most prominent chiropractic colleges to this day.

Chiropractic care has only recently gained a wide degree of acceptance and respectability. For years the American Medical Association worked to discredit the profession but in 1976 Chester Wilk and four other chiropractors filed a lawsuit for restraint of trade. After 14 years of legal battles a federal court ruled against the AMA, finding that they had engaged in an illegal activity, the use of propaganda against chiropractic.

It requires four or five years of study at an accredited chiropractic college to become a doctor of chiropractic. Each person must also pass national board and all state exams in order to practice. There are also individual state licensing requirements in order to be a chiropractor. Anyone interested in beginning chiropractic treatment should research their state's requirements and the background of a potential healthcare professional along with the education and training of any chiropractor they're considering for therapy.

Chiropractic care is one of the few CAM therapies frequently covered by insurance. The 2002 federal survey on the use of complementary and alternative medicine in America found that 19.9% had used chiropractic care at some time in their life and 7.5% had used it in the prior 12 months. In the 2007 survey chiropractic use in the previous 12 months had jumped to 8.6% but the category had been combined with osteopathic manipulation.

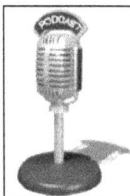

Dr. Kurt Wood is the Executive Dean for Clinic Affairs at Palmer College of Chiropractic in Davenport, Iowa, the first school of chiropractic care in the world. Discover all of the health benefits from this unique American style of therapy and what "pops" during treatment.

www.amerchiro.org

USER COMMENTS:

- If you've ever found yourself on your hands and knees in pain you probably already know how effective chiropractic care can be. Whether it's too much yard work or simply "zigging when you should've zagged" there is nothing like the pain of nerves in the spine!
- Chiropractors will begin with X-rays and then a careful examination of your entire back. If conditions warrant an adjustment then they'll usually massage the back with a machine to

relax the muscles so they'll move more easily. Then they'll hold your feet together to see the length of your legs as a measuring tool for the structure of your spine. It's amazing how they can find each joint that is out of place by your legs, but apparently the stiffness of back muscles changes the relationship of the leg length.

♦ Adjustments can be made manually in different styles or by the use of a device. The 'Activator' is one of the most common tools to deliver consistent pressure at a precise location. It's not uncommon to get a little of both depending on your situation and needs.

♦ Today chiropractors are expanding into new technology like spinal decompression tables and even cold lasers to promote spine health. All too often they'll prescribe wellness to keep you out of trouble in the first place.

COLONIC HYDROTHERAPY IRRIGATION also Colonic Irrigation
or Colonic Hydrotherapy

Colonic Hydrotherapy Irrigation, also called a **Colonic** or **Colonic Hydrotherapy,** is similar to an enema. Small amounts of water are frequently mixed with minerals, enzymes or herbs and introduced into the colon using a medically-approved, class II colon hydrotherapy device. Either disposable speculums or gravity-fed systems may be used. The fluid is released from the colon after a short period and the process is repeated several times during the 40-45 minute procedure.

Colonics are often recommended as part of an alternative treatment program to remove toxins from the body which result from processed foods, pesticides and other unhealthy intake. The process has been used since ancient times to treat constipation but current popularity may be due to the late Max Gerson who passed away in 1959. The German physician believed that coffee enemas eliminate poisons and offered a legitimate treatment for cancer. Today colonics and coffee enemas are often used by cancer patients to speed up the removal of radiation and chemotherapy toxins from their bodies.

Caution is advised with this process since there have been cases of medical complications from unsafe or unsanitary practices. Right now it is only regulated in some states; please review the training and certification of your practitioner along with your state requirements. The International Association of Colon HydroTherapy offers standards and certification.

`www.i-act.org`

USER COMMENTS:

♦ When I was an Air Force pilot doing high-altitude work I trained my body not to defecate so I could fly the 12-hour missions without having to go to the bathroom. At that time I was only having bowel movements every three or four days, sometimes once a week. My doctor said that's just the way it is and prescribed laxatives. Once I retired I discovered colonic hydrotherapy and it's been incredible to get my body functioning again normally. It's a great feeling to be able to go to the bathroom regularly!

CRANIOSACRAL THERAPY (CST) also Cranial Osteopathy and Craniopathy

Craniosacral Therapy or CST is based on the belief that all living tissues have a motion of life which produces rhythmic impulses. This "Breath of Life" was discovered by osteopath Dr. William Sutherland more than 100 years ago. He realized that cranial bones were designed to provide a small amount of motion which he compared to the motion of gills on a fish. These movements involve a network of tissues and fluids at the core of the human body such as spinal fluid, fluid surrounding the brain and the central nervous system. The ability of cells and tissues to express this primary motion is a vital feature for determining our general health.

There are at least three different rhythms in this "primary respiratory system", each with its own rate of vibration and pulse. These pulses are identified as: the cranial rhythmic impulse; the mid-tide and the long tide. Practitioners feel or "listen" through their hands to the patient's body rhythms to detect any patterns of congestion or restriction. They then apply gentle pressure to improve the functioning of the central nervous system so the body can better heal itself.

Manipulation of the skull has been practiced for thousands of years, going back to Egypt, India and Peru. Dr. Sutherland began to teach his therapeutic techniques to remove restrictions in this motion to other osteopaths in the 1930s. It is referred to as craniosacral osteopathy and it is still taught today.

The most common form of craniosacral therapy was developed in the 1970s by Dr. John E. Upledger. His technique resulted from his research at Michigan State University and he began teaching his full-body form of therapy to non-osteopaths, making it much more widely available. By 2009 the Upledger Institute had taught more than 100,000 practitioners in more than 50 countries around the world.

SomatoEmotional Release is a process developed by John Upledger that expands on the concepts of his CST. It's a process that helps to rid the mind and body of residual effects of a past trauma. "Soma" is Greek for "body" so it can be seen as psychotherapy for the body's memories. Such emotional trauma stored in the body can inhibit structural release so it is a complementary technique to CST.

Craniopathy began as chiropractic craniopathy in the 1920s by M.B. Dejarnette, D.C., D.O. as Sacro Occipital Technique. By 1968 he felt his system was sufficiently developed and began teaching craniopathy to the chiropractic profession.

A newer variation based on cranial osteopathy is **Biodynamic Craniosacral Therapy**. This style takes a whole-person approach to healing and the inter-connections of mind, body and spirit.

There is also a type of massage referred to as craniosacral so it's best to check the training and qualifications of your therapist. You could be getting simply a head massage instead of therapy.

In the U.S. the process has a variety of licensing requirements so check your local regulations.

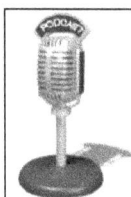

Dr. Lisa Upledger has been a CST practitioner for 28 years and is a certified therapist and instructor at the Upledger Institute. She is also the wife of Dr. John E. Upledger, DO, OMM, the creator of CranioSacral Therapy and the founder of the Upledger Institute.

www.upledger.com, www.sorsi.com, www.craniosacraltherapy.org

USER COMMENTS:

♦ This feels amazing when it's done right, like your brain is being centered. I feel my sinuses start working again and there is a sense of relaxation that flows through my entire body. It literally feels like your body is unwinding from all of the tension. It also leaves you with a sense of wholeness, like you're back to square one being yourself again. Good stuff but I've found a wide range of techniques. Some therapists really know what they're doing and some are just doing a gentle scalp massage.

♦ I experienced this as a very gentle subtle form of healing. The practitioner did touch me but the touch was very light. My legs were gently manipulated. There were times when I was asked to tune into my body and give feedback about what I was experiencing. It was deeply relaxing. I felt as though I was floating.

DIGESTIVE HEALTH THERAPY

There are several different facets of **Digestive Health Therapy**. First there is the general health of the five parts of the digestive tract and its estimated 10,000 different organisms. The small intestine is 15 to 20 feet long and that's where most digestion and absorption of food takes place. Food has always been medicine (remember chicken soup?) and herbal medicine today offers unique advantages for treatment of the digestive system. While there are almost as many self-help books as there are supplements today, the services of a skilled herbalist may be beneficial in diagnosing individual dietary requirements.

There are also specialized fields of Digestive Health Therapy. **Enzymes** or **Enzymatic Therapy** are the biggest area because they're required for almost all chemical activity in the body from digestion, to building bones, for repairing tissues, purifying blood and aiding in detoxification. They are reported to be beneficial for many degenerative diseases by reducing inflammation. Enzymes are reduced in our food today due to processing so the addition of natural food enzymes, corrective dietary habits and whole food supplements in the diet can improve health by improving the digestive system.

Pioneering research into the importance of enzymes goes back more than 50 years with the work of biochemist Dr. Edward Howell. Today we know there are different types of enzymes: dietary; digestive; systemic and metabolic. Dietary enzymes are found in all natural unprocessed foods and aid in the digestion and breakdown of that food. Digestive enzymes are produced by the pancreas and secreted into the stomach and small intestines to aid food enzymes in the digestive process by pre-digesting foods. Metabolic enzymes are produced by the liver and control most chemical reactions in the cells. Systemic enzymes act as catalysts to start and stop chemical reactions such as immune function and hormone balance. Unlike other enzymes these must pass through the stomach to be released into the blood stream.

`www.americanherbalistsguild.com`

USER COMMENTS:

♦ Most people don't realize that those self-help products you find at the health food store can also do a great deal of harm. I took a product to cleanse Candida out of my digestive system (being so very well self-diagnosed) and it worked great the first time. I had no symptoms for a year and felt the best I had in ages. However when I tried the same product again the entire digestive tract went haywire. Nothing I've tried worked and eventually I ended up at the Mayo Clinic.

♦ It's taken a lot of time to rebuild the enzymes and thousands of chemical reactions in my digestive system. The natural balance of this entire flora isn't known to current science and it is such a complicated system you really need to proceed with caution and care. Even when under the supervision of a medical doctor or herbalist exercise extreme caution because you'll be the one to suffer through the trial-and-error of correcting your digestive tract!

DOULA

Doula means the continuous emotional and physical support for women during labor and early postpartum so they can experience satisfying childbirth and postpartum events. The term "doula" describes a woman serving other women. Dr. Marshall Klaus noticed in 1967 that many parents of premature babies were having difficulty adjusting, partly because standard medical practice at that time did not allow mothers into the premature nursery until immediately before discharge. Dr. John Kennell joined with Dr. Klaus to study bonding and their work was instrumental to opening nurseries to parents and to allow parents of normal, full-term babies to be with infants during the first moments after birth.

In the late 1980s and early 1990s, researchers found that women who had used doulas had shorter labors and fewer caesarean births. Recent research shows women who have doula support also have increased rates of breastfeeding, more positive mother-infant relationships and greater satisfaction with their birth experience.

Doulas support families emotionally to help them feel comfortable with the experience. DONA® International was started in 1992 by Drs. Klaus, Kennel along with Phyllis Klaus C.S.W., M.F.C.C., Penny Simkin PT and Annie Kennedy to promote doula care. Today there are nearly 6,000 members worldwide. The association provides training and certification.

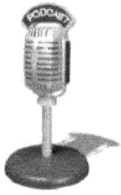

Women are choosing to have a Doula at their side during and after childbirth today and medical research shows there are tremendous benefits for both mother and baby. I spoke with Susan Tofflon, President of DONA International the oldest and largest Doula organization, about women serving women. Susan is also a certified childbirth educator, a DONA certified birth doula and birth Doula trainer.

www.dona.org

USER COMMENTS:

- My doula was indispensable. She helped me move from one position to the other, whispered encouragement in my ear, taught me how to moan lowly and loved me in a time of great need. This resulted in a safe, and quick, natural birth with no drugs and no interventions.

- She acted as an advocate for me. Physically, when I was ready to push, I was shaking badly. She knew little tricks of rubbing my toes that would keep my jaw from chattering. She took photographs, so we didn't have to worry about that. When I finally asked for the epidural, I was nervous about it, but she supported me and did not make me feel guilty at all for getting pain relief. It was just very reassuring to have someone with so much knowledge there, and to have a kind and warm spirit to help us through the whole experience.

EAR CANDLING

Ear Candling is a simple, safe way of removing excess wax and toxins from inside the ears. The process has been used for thousands of years in Egypt, Tibet, India, China, by American Indians and European healers. Today it's used by Amish, in Europe and by others interested in natural healing techniques. It's also called Thermo-Auricular Therapy and Ear Coning.

Originally the straws used in the process were made of pottery clay carved to create a downward spiral of heated air which would carry the smoke of herbs into the ear. The flow also creates a vacuum inside the cone to draw out excess waste and impurities. Today a wide straw of unbleached cotton cloth coated in wax or other material is used to create a vacuum to draw excess ear wax and toxins into the straw in a 30-45 minute process.

The procedure is done with the client lying on their side with a towel wrapped around the ear. The practitioner gently places the narrow end of the cone into the entrance of the ear canal. A paper plate or other collection device is placed at the middle of the candle to collect the melting wax. When the candle is lit the convection process draws the warmed and softened ear waxes up and into the straw bringing out any impurities, toxins or allergens. As the candle burns it's normal to hear crackling and hissing. Many people report the warmth provides a soothing and relaxing experience.

There are many different types of ear candles. Some are made with different types of oils or herbs in the wax for different effects. For example, Biosun candles are very popular in Europe because they do not have any chemical pesticide & fungicidal residues and carry the prestigious CE mark (93/42-EEC class 11a) for medical devices in Europe. Food and Drug Administration regulations prohibit ear candles from being sold or advertised in America as medical devices.

There is a wide range of training for practitioners; some simply have started practicing after being patients. CAUTION is advised since there have been reports of burns and damage to ears from inexperienced therapists and improper use of materials. Also do not use this process if you have a punctured ear drum or other injury to the ear.

www.earcandling.com,
http://www.time.com/time/magazine/article/0,9171,997230,00.html

USER COMMENTS:

- My daughter and I do ear candling on each other because it's so easy. It's a warm and delightful feeling and it does wonders for my sinus headaches and allergies.

- I had been having vertigo for two months; the day after the ear candling session, it was gone. I had a directional hearing problem in my left ear that was also alleviated after the session.

- I've had problems with my ears since my youth. I remember having several ear infections as a boy and as I grew up, I noticed moderate changes and discomfort in my ears throughout my adult life. The ear candling session immediately alleviated the wax build-up. Right away there was a noticeable improvement in my hearing.

> **TIP**
>
> If a Forest of Symptoms/ has you lost/then find your way out/ at any cost./ If you can't see/ the forest for the trees/finding the source/will be the key./ Then with great ease/matching a therapy/you'll find is a breeze.

EGOSCUE®

Egoscue® is a therapy system for posture alignment that involves a series of stretches, gentle Esgoscue® exercises (egoscuecises) and sometimes weightlifting. It is designed to strengthen specific muscles to bring the body into proper alignment and functioning and eliminate pain.

Pete Egoscue is an anatomical physiologist and author of *PAIN FREE - A Revolutionary Method for Stopping Chronic Pain* and co-author of *The Egoscue Method of Health Through Motion*. Suffering a hip injury while serving with the Marines he developed his program to resolve his own pain and began teaching others his techniques in 1978.

The program is designed specifically for each client to relieve pain without manipulation. To begin the Egoscue® therapist evaluates the client's posture then examines the walk and the range of motion to determine where the pain and problem is located. The focus is on straightening before strengthening. The exercise series may be on the floor or sitting and time required can vary from 15 to 90 minutes. Exercises may also use the Egoscue® Multi-Positioning Tower and Multi-Slant Board.

The therapy is available at 25 clinics around the world, at traveling clinics, with the Egoscue® Home Video and Webcam Program and the Egoscue Direct™ Video Conferencing program to link for consultations with Egoscue® therapists over the Internet.

Training to become an Approved Provider of the ePete Postural Software can be completed in just 30 days at the Eposcue® University. To deliver the Postural Therapy to the public as a certified PAS requires a year of education and training.

www.egoscue.com

ENERGY MEDICINE

The new science of **Energy Medicine** or **Electrotherapy** is based on the scientific discovery of a new circulatory system in the human body for electrical energy. This process is remarkably similar to the meridian concepts of Traditional Chinese Medicine.

This new perspective on energy in the human body was developed by internationally renowned Swedish radiologist and surgeon Dr. Bjorn E. W. Nordenstrom and published in *Biologically Closed Electrical Circuits* (1983). Beginning in the mid-1950s Dr. Nordenstrom noticed radiating patterns around cancer tumors on chest X-rays which he called corona structures because they reminded him of the sun's corona. Additional study revealed fluctuating electrical charges within the tumors. This led to the discovery of a new type of system, an electrical circuit that involves the transportation of ions and electrons throughout the body. This circulating current helps maintain the body's equilibrium and healing processes by influencing cellular structure and function.

Blood plasma and interstitial fluid are examples of media capable of conducting current while blood vessel walls, cells and membranes surrounding interstitial spaces provide insulation to the surroundings. In other words, they're insulated electric cables providing communication within the body through electromagnetic signaling. These flowing electrical charges found in the body resemble the "yin and yang" concepts and the flow of Chi discovered 5,000 years ago in ancient China.

The editor of The American Institute of Stress, Paul J. Rosch, M.D., F.A.C.P. wrote in his review of the 1983 book that "...he has demonstrated how specific DC microcurrents that restore ion electricity balance can be utilized to treat metastic lung cancer and other malignancies with amazing success, and his therapeutic triumphs have now been replicated by others in thousands of patients." Following a report by Dr. Tim Johnson on ABC's *20/20* program, host Barbara Walters expressed amazement at this medical breakthrough. More than 12,000 cancer patients around the world have now successfully been treated with electrochemical therapy (EChT) using Dr. Nordenstrom's BCEC concepts.

I call it Star Trek medicine.

There have only been a few limited trials being conducted in America. In what may be one of the most fundamental paradigm shifts in medicine since William Harvey discovered blood circulation 350 years ago, America has taken a back seat in research. Unable to secure funding and support in America, Dr. Nordenstrom was welcomed by China to continue his research. The current five year survival rates for liver cancer are reported to be about 15% in China compared to 5% in the U.S. where they're treated with conventional therapies. In 2001, Dr. Nordenstrom received the International Scientific and Technological Cooperation Award from the People's Republic of China for his work.

EChT treatment is available in Germany, China and other countries. Costs are reported to be in the $7,500 (U.S.) range with treatment taking up to two weeks.

The fundamental premise of this new field of Electrotherapy is wound healing because it artificially enhances the body's natural healing process. The technique is being used for vision treatments and other health problems today.

The International Association for Biologically Closed Electric Circuits in Medicine and Biology (IABC) was founded in 1993 for the development of electrotherapeutic, thermotherapeutic and magnetotherapeutic techniques, along with conventional therapies, for the treatment of health problems including cancer.

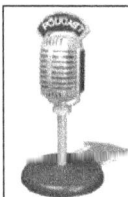

> The 51st podcast was with George O'Clock, Ph.D., former president of the IABC and author of *ELECTROTHERAPEUTIC DEVICES: Principles, Design and Applications* about Nordenstrom, Becker and the new era of medicine using BCEC.

www.iabc.readywebsites.com/page/page/623957.htm

ENVIRONMENTAL MEDICINE

Environmental Medicine is a new perspective based on a traditional approach to health care. The process decreases the focus on the disease and increases the awareness of the causes, frequently the environment of the person. It is a comprehensive, proactive, patient-centric approach to medical care dedicated to the management and prevention of environmental problems. In contrast, mainstream medicine often treats the environment and diet as benign factors in the health equation even though there continues to be explosive growth in the occurrence of more complex and chronic diseases in America.

The new model of environmental medicine employs both Western and Eastern concepts with an appreciation that human beings are constantly coping and adapting to a dynamic environment. **Homeodynamic functioning** refers to the maintenance of health as an active process with optimal health being a balance of physical, neuro-cognitive, psychological and social wellbeing. Stressors to this balance range from organic substances like molds and pollens to man-made chemicals and physical factors like heat, cold, noise and various types of radiation. Treatments for each patient must be customized because each person is a unique organism. Initial appointments frequently require an hour or more to do the detective work necessary to develop a complete picture of the patient and their body's total stress load.

Treatment begins with patient education about the nature of the illness. Therapies may include customized diets, nutritional supplements, immunotherapies, psychotherapies, detoxification therapies, drugs and possibly even surgery.

The American Academy of Environmental Medicine was formed in 1965. It provides the only comprehensive continuing education and training program for MDs and DOs in environmental medicine. The American and International Boards of Environmental Medicine are independent groups which grant board certification and establish educational and training criteria. As with all therapies, it is recommended that customers research and review the training and qualifications of their providers.

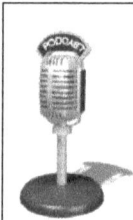	Dr. Amy Dean, Board Member of the American Academy of Environmental Medicine and Chairman of its Public Relations Committee, talked about how many chronic and acute health problems that fail to respond to mainstream medicine may actually be caused by our environment. Listen to some of the ways to protect your health from environmental damage every day. Dr. Dean is board certified in both Internal Medicine and Holistic Medicine.

`www.aaemonline.org, www.aehf.com, www.niehs.nih.gov`

FELDENKRAIS METHOD®

The **Feldenkrais Method**® is a process of educating the body which expands the assortment of movements, enhances awareness, improves function and enables people to express themselves more fully. It is very popular with dancers, musicians and artists. It can be used by anyone who wants to reconnect with their natural ability to move, think and feel. It is also effective at improving movement-related pain and functioning in cases of stroke or cerebral palsy. It is not a massage, bodywork, or necessarily a therapeutic technique, it's a learning process. In contrast to other structural integration therapies the Feldenkrais Method® does not adhere to an idealized form but relies on the internal wisdom of the body to find what is right.

A core belief of the Feldenkrais Method® is that improving the ability to move can improve one's overall well being. It is based on principles of physics, biomechanics and an empirical understanding of learning and human development. The Method is an educational system that uses movement and awareness as the primary method for learning and its purpose is to give greater functional awareness, defined as the interaction of the person with the outside world or the self with the environment. By teaching people how their whole body cooperates in any movement helps them live their lives more fully, efficiently and comfortably.

The Feldenkrais Method® is expressed in two parallel forms. **Awareness Through Movement**® lessons are organized around a particular function and normally last 30-60 minutes. There are hundreds of hours of these verbally-directed movement sequences which evolve from comfortable, easy movements into movements of greater range and complexity. **Functional Integration®** is a hands-on form of tactile, kinesthetic communication. The practitioner communicates to the student how they organize their body by gentle touching and movement which shows how to move in more expanded and functional ways. The lesson is usually performed lying on a table designed specifically for the work but it can also be done with the student in sitting or standing positions.

Moshe Pinhas Feldenkrais moved to Tel Aviv in 1954 and made his living for the first time solely by teaching his Functional Integration method. In the late 1950s Feldenkrais presented his work in Europe and The United States. In the mid-1960s he published *Mind and Body* and *Bodily Expression*. In 1967, he published *Improving the Ability to Perform*, titled *Awareness through Movement* in its 1972 English language edition.

The Feldenkrais Guild® of North America provides accredited Training Programs which are required to be certified, to become members of FGNA, and to use its service marked terms for The Method. Feldenkrais®, Feldenkrais Method®, Awareness Through Movement® and Functional Integration® are registered service marks of the Feldenkrais Guild® of North America. In the 2007 federal survey 96 people responded they'd used it in the previous 12 months but it was such a small response it was a 0.0%.

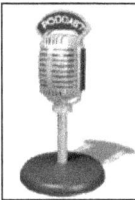

MaryBeth Smith, the Director of the Feldenkrais® Center in Houston, Texas and a Certified Feldenkrais® Practitioner explained that the therapy developed by Dr. Moshe Feldenkrais is widely regarded as the most gentle of the structural integration therapies.

www.feldenkrais.com, www.feldenkrais-method.org

USER COMMENTS:

♦ The Method creates a smoothness of motion that is absolutely wonderful. The motions can be so small and subtle that you don't feel a thing, until the next day. Then you can be sore as hell! It's amazing how such miniscule changes in posture or motion can have such big repercussions in your whole body.

♦ Feldenkrais is a lot less invasive than Rolfing and it's focused more on connecting the mind to the body so the muscles move the way they're supposed to, it's a much more subtle process. After a session I usually walk a couple of blocks just to rediscover my body and it's amazing how much lighter it feels and how much more fluid my movements are.

♦ As an aging ex-jock, nursing bad knees and shoulders, Functional Integration® and Awareness Through Movement® work helps me develop insight into how my body operates and how it compensates for old injuries. With a more solid understanding of 'what is,' I can start to make intelligent choices about how I want to move, sit, stand and just function.

FLOATATION THERAPY

Floatation Therapy, originally known as sensory deprivation, was created in 1954 by Dr. John C. Lilly, an American neurophysiologist and psychoanalyst. He expected to learn about the brain in sleep states but discovered that the mind becomes even more active when deprived of outside stimulation. It's also been called **Restricted Environmental Stimulation Technique** (REST) since the 1970s. The process produces profound relaxation which allows the mind and body to regenerate natural energy without interference. There are similarities between this process and some forms of meditation.

There are two major types of floatation devices, wet or dry. Clients float directly in the water in the wet version, but rest on a sheet of plastic on top of the water in the dry version. Most floatation tanks measure about eight feet long and four feet wide and contain just enough very warm water to float. The water is loaded with salts and minerals making it nearly impossible to sink. Clients will shower before and after each session which may last from one to two hours. There are variations depending on customer preferences such as complete darkness or having a little light and having the tank completely closed or having the lid left open slightly. Some people prefer total quiet while others request soft music or even self-hypnosis tapes for losing weight or to stop smoking. There is usually a 2-way microphone built into the tank for communication and safety.

The deep relaxation produced by this environment has beneficial effects on the body, primarily in increased healing capacity. There are also psychological benefits connected with the process. By reducing stress it's been useful in the treatment of obsessive and addictive behaviors. Floatation tanks may be found in health clubs and spas or purchased for home use.

There are warnings about this type of therapy is you have a history of psychological disorders, especially claustrophobia.

www.samadhitank.com

USER COMMENTS:

♦ This is how I feel about floating: I am light and expanded within a safe cocoon of space. It is filling, simple and complete. Mainly I know I'm doing something very good for me. It is a healing, an acknowledgement, a growing. It is a good thing.

♦ So, there I was in darkness and silence, floating. It was as black as black could be, silent as a tomb. The water was so buoyant that I floated right on the surface, feeling as secure as I would on a rubber mattress and a lot more comfortable. I soon felt more relaxed than I ever had in my life, free of gravity, floating in warm, silent peaceful space, alone with my mind. Then I realized that I no longer had a body, but the discovery didn't upset me, I didn't even bother to wiggle my fingers—the perfect repose of floating, the stillness of silence was too sublime, too euphoric to disturb. And it occurred to me that all sorts of interesting, exciting things were happening in this black, empty nothingness.

GERMAN NEW MEDICINE

In 1978 Dr. Ryke Geerd Hamer, M.D. was head internist in the oncology clinic at the University of Munich, Germany when his son was shot and killed. Months later he developed cancer and he thought that the shock he'd received might be the cause of the cancer. His research showed that all of his cancer patients had also experienced some type of major upset prior to their cancers. He also learned that "conflict shock" could be traced to a particular part of the brain and a correlation with the organs of the entire body. Dr. Hamer called his findings "The Five Biological Laws of the New Medicine" which offer a new understanding of the natural healing process of diseases.

To honor his son, Dr. Hamer called such an unanticipated stressful event a Dirk Hamer Syndrome or DHS. But a DHS isn't just a psychological event, it's really a biological conflict that needs to be understood on the basis of evolution. It's an experience which we were not prepared. This is the First Biological Law.

The Second Biological Law says that the resolution of the conflict progresses in two stages. The first or conflict-active stage says that the entire organism is dealing with the conflict. This features sleep disturbances and reduction of appetite which are necessary to process and handle the unexpected situation. The second stage has the organism shifting to a healing mode with renewed appetite.

The Third Biological Law states that the cell loss or proliferation in the brain following a DHS are a meaningful part of the biological system. The Fourth Biological Law says that microbes don't cause diseases but instead play a critical role during the healing phase. The Fifth Biological Law says that Nature is orderly and that nothing is meaningless or malignant. Every so-called disease is a part of a Significant Biological Special Program of Nature

http://learninggnm.com/home.html

HALOTHERAPY

Similar to the salt caves of Eastern Europe, salt air inhalation therapy is an easy-to-use drug-free method that eases symptoms of respiratory problems (halo = salt). Salt therapy simply means sitting in a room coated with salt crystals and pumped full of salt-laden air but instead of a cave patrons today experience comfy lounge chairs and flat-screen TVs. Halotherapy is said to improve symptoms of allergy, asthma and skin conditions like psoriasis. Normally the walls and ceilings of a therapy room are salt-coated, and grains are often scattered a few inches deep on the floor so kids can play in it like it was a sandbox.

There is very little research available but a 2006 study in the *New England Journal of Medicine* found that inhaling hypertonic saline improved lung function in people with cystic fibrosis. Also in 2006, a study in the *European Respiratory Journal* of cigarette smokers found that inhaling aerosolized salt temporarily improved smoking-related symptoms such as coughing and mucus production.

https://en.wikipedia.org/wiki/Halotherapy

HELLERWORK STRUCTURAL INTEGRATION

Hellerwork Structural Integration combines deep-tissue structural bodywork, movement education and dialogue to restore the body's natural balance. It's based on the concept that the body, mind and spirit are inseparable so they must be treated as a whole.

Therapy is customized to each individual but built on a standard 11-step series. Most of the work done in the one-hour sessions takes place on a massage table but sitting or standing work may also be included. The process first works with the connective tissue to realign the muscle-skeleton system to restore balance and ease of motion. Movement education trains the person to move with minimum effort. The dialogue process explores how thoughts, beliefs and attitudes impact the body. Hellerwork feels like slow deep pressure that is followed by a sensation of release. Clients may need to make slow motions while the practitioner guides the tissue. Practitioners are trained in the amount of pressure to use, speed and technique but sensations may vary from pleasure to mild, temporary discomfort based on the condition of the tissue.

Hellerwork believes that everyone is innately healthy but to maximize your health you must develop deeper experience with your movement, the integrity of your body and your relationship with yourself and your world.

Joseph Heller was born in Poland in 1940 but came to the U.S. at age 16. He studied with Ida Rolf, the originator of Rolf Structural Integration, becoming a Rolfer in 1972. He also studied Structural Patterning from Judith Ashton. He became the first president of the Rolf Institute in 1975 and continued studying with Ida Rolf until 1978 when he left the Institute to create a new type of bodywork called Hellerwork.

Training and certification is done by the American Hellerwork Structural Integration Association. As a type of bodywork it requires massage licensing in most states. Please check the training, qualifications and licensing of your practitioner before beginning any type of bodywork therapy.

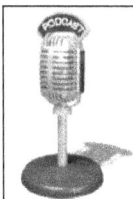

My interview with Joseph Heller, the creator of Hellerwork, covered everything from how he started as an engineer in the space program to the evolution of Hellerwork today. Hellerwork integrates the whole person by combining bodywork with movement education and dialogue in each themed session.

www.hellerwork.com

USER COMMENTS:

♦ Hellerwork has been the least amount of effort, the least amount of time, the least amount of money for the greatest amount of benefit of anything I have ever done.

♦ I was a professional hockey player for 20 years ... (after) Hellerwork ... my posture was better, joints moved easier, I could breathe easier and this was only after a few sessions.

♦ As an old nurse, my back has taken me on a magical mystery tour of alternative health... Hellerwork helped me the most, not just in simple symptom relief (though there is no finer bodywork system) but in the process of developing a relationship with my poor, abused and ignored body. Since completing the series... I have enjoyed happy good health, and a two way communication with my lumbar spine, which in a friendly way reminds me when I need to pay it more attention.

HERBAL BODY WRAP

Herbal Body Wraps were created to shrink the size of the body, offering a slimmer body very quickly. There are a wide variety of products and treatments available using an assortment of ingredients. There are self-help products to use at home and treatments available at spas or from your local massage therapist.

Body Wraps claim to work by shrinking fat cells by assisting them to release toxins, firming and toning the skin. Others claim that success lies in its ability to compact the body. Clay wraps are said to function as a poultice to draw impurities from the body. Skeptics say it simply dehydrates the body so any size reduction is temporary and will be lost as soon as the body is hydrated with fluids again.

The process may use a proprietary blend of herbs and minerals, sea vegetation, sea salt, sea mud, aloe vera, amino acids and other ingredients. Cloth strips are soaked in the solution and wrapped around portions of the body or the entire body which makes you look like an Egyptian mummy. If only portions of the body are wrapped then trapped wastes may simply move from one part of the body to another instead of being eliminated. When you're properly wrapped in cloth strips you are then wrapped in plastic or wear a rubberized outfit to retain body heat, and simply lie in your tub at home or on a table at the spa for about an hour.

In general, licensed massage therapists can do body wraps for muscle relaxation and rehabilitation in most states and estheticians can do body wraps for the purpose of beautifying the skin. Regulations vary so please check with your appropriate state licensing agency. There are also a variety of products designed for home us available in stores and on the Internet.

http://www.webmd.com/beauty/spa/body-wraps-what-to-expect

USER COMMENTS:

♦ Thank you for The Body Wrap! In just one month I am 36" smaller, my body looks and feels great! My skin is much smoother and I have much more energy. Keep up the good work!

♦ When I first discovered The Body Wrap about 3 years ago, I had lost some weight - from 200 lbs. down to 179. Also, over this period my weight was down to 130 lbs. and never during the weight loss did my skin appear baggy or loose. I was very pleased with the smooth, toned appearance of my skin. I am very pleased with the results I have experienced and look forward to my wraps.

HIJAMA WET CUPPING THERAPY

Hijama is a uniquely Muslim style of treatment which can benefit anyone. While any physician or acupuncturist can perform wet cupping only a Muslim can administer Hijama Therapy because they will be following the Islamic rules. In the Muslim religion the divine nature and high status given to Hijama is reflected in the fact that Muhammad said that the Angels told him and his

Ummah (Nation) to practice Cupping. The technique claims to boost the circulatory and immune systems and cleanse and detoxify the body. It can be used for headaches, joint pain, pulled muscles, poor circulation and other health problems.

There are several steps to the process. First a small plastic cup is placed over the area to be treated and a vacuum created to pull the toxins to the surface. After a few minutes the cup is removed and lots of small cuts are placed over the area and the cup is replaced with renewed vacuum. After several more minutes the cup collects an amount of a gelatinous blood which is carefully removed as the cup is taken away. This process removes the toxins and other materials causing discomfort.

http://hijamanation.com/

HULDA CLARK PROTOCOL

This process consists of a combination of methods designed to detox and cleanse the body so the immune system can function properly thereby curing a variety of diseases. The **Hulda Clark Protocol** was based on her own biofeedback research. Using her Syncrometer device that she believed could detect the causes of cancer, HIV and other diseases using her process she could then cleanse the body with her Zapper device. This technique is based on the concept that all living thing have their own frequency including viruses, parasites and even toxins.

Dr. Hulda Regehr Clark, Ph.D., N.D. wrote 5 books on cancer, a book on HIV/AIDS and a book on illnesses in general. A Canadian born in 1928 she received her doctorate degree in physiology from the University of Minnesota. Her studies were focused on biophysics and cell physiology during her career. She passed away in 2009.

Dr. Clark's Syncrometer is an audio oscillator circuit that is supposed to detect resonance in a manner similar to a radio. It is used to scan the body for parasites, viruses, bacteria and toxins. Her Zapper is a battery-operated device that generates positive, off-set frequencies to kill all bacteria, viruses and parasites simultaneously in less than seven minutes. Treatments often include a series of Zapper sessions to eliminate the entire chain of contamination in the body. Combined with other features of her protocol including the Zappicator, Sonicator, Ozonator and Colloidal Silver to sterilize food and water and her herbal cleanses the process is supposed to clean the body and permit the immune system to perform. Her therapy also places great importance on pure and potent vitamins, herbal supplements along with high-quality food products. The 21-day cleansing protocol is even used on advanced cancer.

As with many CAM therapies FDA regulations do not permit Dr. Clark's Zapper to be sold for medical use on people or animals; however it can be purchased for water treatment or as an experimental device. There are also plans available on the Internet to build your own devices.

www.drhuldaclark.org/

HYDROGEN PEROXIDE THERAPY

Hydrogen Peroxide (H2O2) Therapy has been used for more nearly a century. One of the earliest reports of the treatment was by Dr. T.H. Oliver in the British Medical Journal (Lancet) in 1920. Since that time it has been the subject of many research studies, many focusing on its use to neutralize free radical chemistry.

Our body naturally produces hydrogen peroxide, it is even used by our immunological system to oxidize foreign invaders. The therapy has many health benefits including treating arthritis because of its ability to supply oxygen to the oxygen-hating organisms that are supposed to cause the condition. Using 35% H2O2 in a cold humidifier can be a beneficial treatment for colds. Hyperoxygenation by hydrogen peroxide is supposed to kill cancer cells according to proponents.

Hydrogen peroxide may be given either orally or by IV drip for medical purposes with intravenous being the more popular method due to the potential for vomiting with the oral method. CAUTION: Any medical use of hydrogen peroxide requires a pure, food-grade type of hydrogen peroxide, a completely different product from the type at the local drug store.

One of the early supporters of the therapy was Dr. Edward Rosenow, a physician and research scientist associated with the Mayo Clinic for several decades. Father Richard Willhelm was the founder of ECHO or the Educational Concern for Hydrogen Peroxide in the 1940s. More recently Charles H. Farr, MD, PhD, was the founder and first president of the International Bio-Oxidative Medical Foundation. The 2003 book *The Many Benefits Of Hydrogen Peroxide* by Dr. David G. Williams offers updated information.

It should be noted that although positive research on this therapy has been done at Baylor Medical Center and other hospitals the FDA continues to aggressively prosecute anyone offering this therapy outside of their strict, research conditions. Clinics in Mexico and Europe do offer the therapy.

`http://www.earthclinic.com/remedies/hydrogen_peroxide.html`

USER COMMENTS:

♦ My patients have enjoyed wonderful results from hydrogen peroxide therapy. I've used the treatment for many different conditions but allergies respond especially well, in many cases relief occurs before the drip has even been completed. It's unfortunate that so many state medical boards are prosecuting doctors for this proven therapy.

HYDROTHERAPY or Hydropathy

Hydrotherapy is using water for health and **hydrothermal therapy** adds temperature, as in hot baths or saunas. This is one of the oldest forms of therapy going back to ancient Greeks. Public communal baths were also part of ancient Rome. China and Japan also had bathing as part of their ancient cultures. Being immersed or doing exercises in water has been a popular therapy in many cultures for thousands of years.

There are many different methods of hydrotherapy including: baths and showers; **colonics**; douches; localized therapies like sitz or foot baths; steam inhalation; hot compresses and body wraps to name just a few. The healing properties of water are based on its mechanical effects (either pressure or jets) or its thermal effects. In addition various herbs or salts may be used to enhance the experience. Heated water in a whirlpool or bath naturally soothes the body while the weightlessness of being in water helps to relieve stress and muscle tension. When pressurized jets are used circulation is boosted helping to release tight muscles. From spas in Europe to thermal springs across America like Hot Springs, Arkansas and Palm Springs, California, hot water therapy has always been popular. These naturally heated hot springs often contain a variety of minerals which are promoted as having special healing powers.

A **sauna**, also called a Turkish or hot air bath, can have temperatures of 120 to 212 degrees with 150 degrees Fahrenheit being the norm. There are also moist air steam baths. In either case, the heat stimulates the body to sweat toxins out through the skin. They also stimulate blood flow, increase heart rate, open airways and promote hormone production. Exposure can range from twenty minutes up to two hours. This is similar to the sweat lodge used by Native American Indian tribes.

Another common type of hydrotherapy is a wrap, either hot or cold. Primarily used as a supportive measure for treating fever and local inflammation, a moistened cloth is wrapped around the body or its affected part and then covered with a dry cloth. If a cool wrap is used to reduce inflammation the process will probably last 45 minutes to an hour. If a warm cloth is used to produce sweating the procedure may last hours.

When using a spa or hot tub a neutral temperature ranging between 92 and 94 degrees is recommended to relieve tension but a higher temperature of 102 to 106 degrees is often suggested if the goal is to relax muscles. Taking a cold shower after a hot bath can be very invigorating!

Please consult your doctor to determine if this type of therapy is suitable for your condition. Many people should avoid this type of therapy. People with diabetes should avoid any hot body wrap but especially to their feet or legs. Immersion in hot baths or using hot saunas is not recommended for diabetics, pregnant women, and people with multiple sclerosis or anyone with abnormally high or low blood pressure. The elderly and children should also exercise caution. Always be sure to drink plenty of water to replace what's been lost!

`http://www.holisticonline.com/hydrotherapy.htm`

USER COMMENTS:

♦ A hot tub is fine and my personal Jacuzzi tub is wonderful after a strenuous day but there is nothing like the full treatment at a spa. I visited Hot Springs, Arkansas to enjoy a real hot spring dip and massage. The water is heated deep in the earth and comes up at 147 degrees so it's mixed with cooler water for comfort. There are ancient American Indian legends about the healing powers of the Valley of the Vapors so in 1832 Congress created the first federally protected area in the national park system for these thermal springs.

There are plenty of choices along Bathhouse Row but we chose the historic Park Hotel which was opened in 1930. History seemed to ooze out of the walls, from Prohibition to visits by President Franklin Roosevelt to modern times. You have your choice of just how hot you want your own hot spring bath. The massage afterwards was short and basic but incredibly relaxing. There are even faucets in the park and along Bathhouse Row so anyone can fill up a jug of this special water to drink. We took home several bottles.

> **TIP**
>
> You'll know when you've found one/by the light that will show/not over your head/in your heart it will glow.

IRIDOLOGY

Iridology is based on the concept that the patterns, colors, and other characteristics of the irises in the eye can be used to diagnose our health. While poets have long said that the eyes are the windows to the soul, iridologists believe they also reflect our health. Scientists will only admit that eye scans are one of the most common biometrics being used for security identification today because like fingerprints no two irises are exactly alike.

The earliest mention of "eye diagnosis" was in the 19th century by a Hungarian physician but the first example of the basic concepts goes back to the 16th century. It was popularized in America during the 1950s by Bernard Jensen, a chiropractor and author of more than 50 books on health and healing.

Using a variety of devices to examine or record the eye, practitioners do not diagnose specific diseases but rather recognize the systems and organs that are healthy and the ones that aren't. The condition and changes of the eyes are said to indicate a tendency towards illnesses or to reflect previous health problems.

The fundamental theory of Iridology is that tissues in the body have a direct effect on the iris of the eye so changes in the body produce changes in the iris. There are at least 20 different maps of the iris recognized by various schools of Iridology, each dividing the iris into approximately 80 to 90 different zones. In addition to a variety of national models around the world of Iridology there is also Physical Iridology, Applied Iridology, the Spiritual Iridology Model and the Rayid Method among many others.

The International Iridology Practitioners Association was founded in 1982 but the name was changed to the International Iridology Practitioners Association in 2000. The IIPA trains and certifies practitioners but there are no official standards of practice in most countries. www.iridologyassn.org

LYPOSSAGE™

Lypossage™ was created by Charles W. Wiltsie III, a licensed massage therapist in Connecticut, to help women lose size without losing weight and help them reduce the appearance of cellulite. He came up with the original idea in 1998 and today Lypossage™ has become part of both the massage therapy and the health and spa industries.

Lypossage™ can be done manually or with the G5 Lypossage™ 3 Zone Massage Machine to improve appearance without liposuction, or to complement cosmetic surgery. Stalled lymphatic fluid can cause unsightly and unwanted bulges so Lypossage™ helps to cleanse the body, improve lymph flow and break up the connective fibers that hold fat in the dimpled areas. It also helps to tone muscles and firm sagging tissues, especially in the lower face and neck area along with the buttocks and upper thighs.

Only professionals trained by Pro-Actif Spa Systems International, its certified Master Trainers or 5 Star Educators may use the trademarked term "Lypossage™".
www.lypossage.net

USER COMMENTS:

♦ As your slogan says, I now feel as good as I look. I have energy now and enjoy spending more time playing with my kids. I now can get a full night's rest without waking up every hour. Best decision that I have made to help improve myself.

♦ I tried everything under the moon to fit into my favorite dress and by the time I completed the Lypossage™ Treatment, the dress was too big!

♦ By age 45, my waistline was almost nonexistent. After just three sessions of Lypossage, I've lost over an inch from hips and waist. More important is an increased energy level and the ability to move my body like I could at age 25! I can't wait to do all 18 sessions.

MANUAL LYMPHATIC DRAINAGE (MLD) also Lymph Drainage Therapy (LDT)

Manual Lymphatic Drainage was created in the early 1930s by Danish scientist Dr. Emil Vodder as a series of massaging motions for the relief of chronic sinus congestion and immune disorders. Later it became a major therapy for the management of Lymphedema, a swelling in the arms and legs caused by the accumulation of lymphatic fluid.

The majority of the lymphatic system is located just below the surface of the skin using body motion to move fluids to the kidneys and liver for elimination. Injury, infection or surgery that removes the lymph nodes can slow or block this flow of fluid resulting in Lymphedema.

MLD uses a range of specialized and rhythmic motions to stimulate the lymphatic vessels. Light sweeping movements promote the flow of lymph into the capillaries near the surface of the skin. Stronger motions push the lymph to flow more deeply into the tissues. There are also specialized MLD movements to soften problem tissues. There are several major styles of this therapy including the Vodder, Foldi, and Leduc or Casley-Smith. Sessions normally last 30 to 60 minutes depending on the patient's condition. Patients can expect an increased need to urinate so they're encouraged to drink plenty of water following a session to replace fluids mobilized by the treatment.

In all cases it is a very specialized type of massage that should only be given by a trained therapist. However once you've been properly taught the techniques you can perform a simplified version of MLD on yourself called **Simple Lymphatic Drainage** (SLD).

A more recent style of treatment was developed by French physician Dr. Bruno Chikly as a direct result of his award-winning research on the lymphatic system. **Lymph Drainage Therapy** (LDT) adds a new level of precision to traditional techniques. Therapists use all of their fingers with a flat hand to simulate gentle, wave-like motions with specific movements. Therapists are able to activate lymph and interstitial fluid circulation with these techniques and stimulate the immune and parasympathetic nervous systems.

As a type of massage therapy all practitioners must be licensed massage therapists. The US National Lymphedema Network cautions anyone taking anticoagulants, congestive heart patients and anyone else who may be sensitive to lymph movement. If you have any questions or concerns please check with your personal physician before beginning this type of therapy.
`www.vodderschool.com, http://www.lymphnet.org/`

USER COMMENTS:

♦ Who knew that a lymph node could be so painful? These are things you didn't even know you had until somebody shows you how important they are to your health. Even an experienced massage therapist with a very light touch can get your attention when they first touch a node or collection/transmission spot and it's full or blocked. Ouch! What's really strange is that your whole body can be fine and just one spot can have a problem … but it's a problem. The good news is that a good massage therapist can get things flowing again quickly and easily. Afterwards you feel lighter, more relaxed and just right again. It's funny how you may not notice that you're not feeling 100% until after you've had a massage with lymph drainage and then you feel 110%.

♦ An experienced therapist can feel the fluids flow underneath their fingers so they can gently unblock the system and getting it moving again. Sometimes there may be little discomfort because the system is working well and the MLD is just sort of a flush. Other times, part of it really needs the help. In any case it's a very beneficial process that helps the body maintain good health.

MĀORI HEALING

Te oomai reia, also called **Māori Healing**, are the traditional healing methods of the Māori, an indigenous people in New Zealand thought to have emigrated from the Hawaiian Islands thousands of years ago. Considered "bush medicine" this information has been passed down orally through the generations by the Māori Tohunga or High Priest/Priestess and the Tohuna, the keepers of the secrets.

To understand the purpose of Māori Healing one must appreciate the four cornerstones of Māori health: taha whānau (family health); taha tinana (physical health); taha hinengaro (mental health) and taha wairua (spiritual health). In the Māori culture they believe that we are spiritual beings having an earthly experience and that we have the ability to use the powers of nature to heal ourselves.

These traditional holistic healing methods include mirimiri (massage) rongoa (herbal treatments) and karakia (spiritual prayer) along with other techniques such as water therapy. The mirimiri is a deep-tissue massage where acupressure is put on the nervous system, tendons, bones and muscles in order to free trapped emotions and energy, a process that can be very painful. The healers also use natural tools including rakau made from certain types of wood, kohatu which are stones and crystals and rongoa which are the natural medicines made from plants, roots and bark. The Māori healer works physically but also in the energy field.

In contrast to many other therapies Māori healers work in a group and it's not unusual to have several healers work with you at the same time. It's not uncommon to have several people being treated in the same room simultaneously. During the session the healers often sing, pray and even laugh to help you to free yourself energetically and emotionally to allow your body to heal itself. Treatments are customized for everyone's personal path to health and peace.

It should be noted that the Māori have on average the poorest health standards of any ethnic group in New Zealand. In 1993 the Ngā Ringa Whakahaere o te Iwi Māori was established to preserve the knowledge of traditional Māori healers. The government continues to work with the Tohunga to involve Māori with modern health practices to offer them the best of both worlds. The New Zealand Public Health & Disability Act 2000 requires the Te Kete Hauora (the Māori Health Directorate) to work with their District Health Boards to work with the Māori to improve their health.

`http://tinyurl.com/4Maori, www.aiohealing.com`

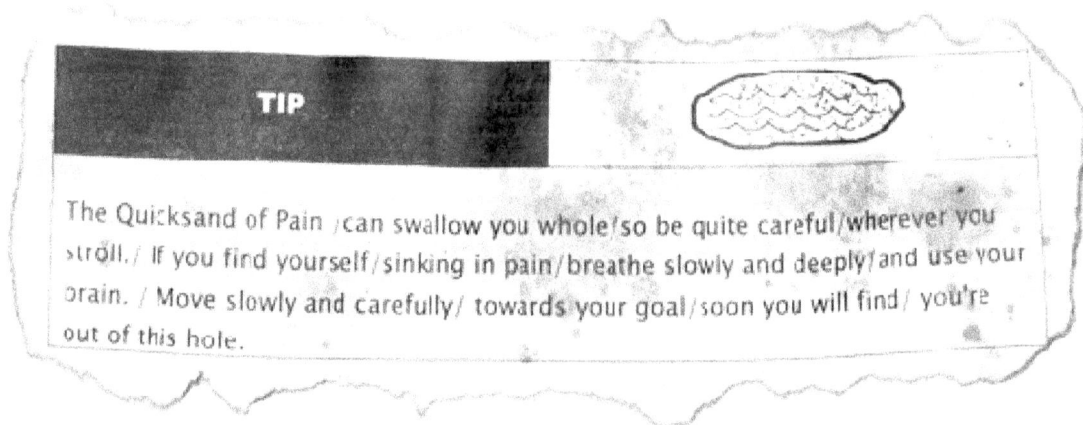

TIP

The Quicksand of Pain / can swallow you whole/ so be quite careful/wherever you stroll. / If you find yourself/ sinking in pain / breathe slowly and deeply/ and use your brain. / Move slowly and carefully/ towards your goal /soon you will find / you're out of this hole.

MASSAGE

A **Massage** is the process of applying pressure, tension, motion, or vibration to the soft tissues of the body. Working on the muscles, tendons, ligaments, joints, connective tissue or lymph system for a positive response can be done manually or with the aid of a device. In addition to just feeling wonderful it can be a form of therapy for all or part of the body, to help injuries heal, relieve stress, improve circulation or to help control pain. It is one of the oldest forms of therapy because it's been used by a variety of cultures for thousands of years.

According to the 2002 survey by the federal government 9.3% of those surveyed reported they'd had a massage at some time in their lives. The report showed that 5.0% said they'd had a massage in the previous 12 months but in the 2007 report the figure increased to 8.3%. The growing popularity may reflect a shift in consumer attitude towards massage from simply a feel-good spa treatment to an effective healing therapy, especially for stress. Massage is also one of the most common types of CAM therapies offered by hospitals.

There are many different types of massage to choose from but there are several basic principles. First, good communication is essential to a beneficial massage. Client and massage therapist need to talk about what's expected before beginning the session. What areas need work or need to be avoided? How much pressure is comfortable? In addition the client's medical history and current physical condition need to be reviewed.

Depending on the type of massage it can involve the client lying on a massage table, sitting in a massage chair, or lying on a pad on the floor. In the U.S. clients are usually unclothed but draped with towels or sheet for warmth and privacy. The massage may be done beginning with the client facing up or down and then reversing for the second half of the session.

The following is a partial list of the different types of massage. Please note that the American Massage Therapy Association began the National Certification Exam in 1992. This exam is often used by states to regulate massage practitioners. Please check with your state's certification agency regarding local laws and regulations for massage therapists. Always remember to ask about your massage therapist's training and experience before beginning a massage.

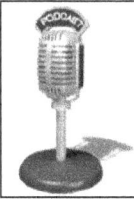

Dr. Leena S. Guptha is the immediate past president of the American Massage Therapy Association and currently Dean of the Massage Therapy program at Lehigh Valley College. You'll enjoy our conversation about this wonderfully relaxing healing therapy.

www.amtamassage.org, www.abmp.com

USER COMMENTS:

♦ The massage experience totally depends on the therapist and what kind of massage you are getting at the moment. From my experience as a practitioner, every massage is a different experience, but always a totally relaxing moment. A massage can take you to Nirvana—to a place of ecstasy—that can totally relax the tension in the muscles. It is very important to drink water after a massage to help get rid of the toxins that the therapist has released. Some people get very relaxed after a massage but others get energized.

BAREFOOT DEEP TISSUE

This technique is a combination of the barefoot styles of the Far East with Western bodywork. Clients normally lie on a floor mat, possibly with pillows or bolsters, and remain clothed. Sessions may last only a few minutes or more than an hour depending on the client's needs and condition. No oil is used because only a small area is worked on at one time. As a result of the therapist being able to apply a wide range of pressure very easily they're able to concentrate more closely on sensing the condition of the tissue being massaged for a more effective treatment. John Harris developed this modality as a deep tissue massage and for working on trigger points regardless of the size of the client.

Chair Massage or Corporate Massage

Perhaps one of the most convenient forms of massage, this technique is done with the client sitting in a special massage chair fully clothed but with restrictions like ties loosened for comfort. This technique focuses on the back, shoulders, neck and arms. Designed to relieve stress and promote circulation it normally lasts less than 25 minutes.

USER COMMENTS:

♦ This is one of the most wonderful innovations for trade shows and conventions! After standing or walking around all day on the concrete floors of a convention hall this type of quick massage can save your back, your legs and your whole body. No wonder there are usually long lines waiting for a chair massage!

♦ My office has been using chair massage services for over a year and a half now and all we can say is we are ALWAYS looking forward to it! I personally would go crazy if we didn't have her here in our office at least once a month. My wish would be to have her here daily...but that's for the company to decide.

Deep Tissue Massage

This type of massage is often used to focus on a specific problem area. The massage therapist begins with a light, easy pressure and then works slowly into the depth of the muscle or soft tissues with gradually increasing pressure. Muscles may tighten if pressure is applied too deeply or quickly, possibly even causing damage, so it's important for the process to be slow and gradual with the comfort of the client in mind. Very little lubricant is used with this technique since it is focused in one small area at a time.

Erotic Massage or Tantra Massage

This very personal type of massage focuses on the genitals to stimulate blood flow and arousal. It is normally practiced by the sexual partner using self-help training materials.

Foot Massage

This localized form of massage uses several different types of motions. Stroking stimulates the blood vessels in the feet and promotes gentle warmth. A slow, easy rotation of the ankle is done to release stress and tension. Pivoting is done by the practitioner using their thumb to rub the toe joint on the bottom of the foot which can wiggle the toe. Toe Pulls are simply a gentle pulling motion applied to each toe which can pop the joint. Kneading the bottom of the foot is often done with the practitioner's fist. A technique called Finger Walking is simply rubbing one spot, usually with the thumb, and then moving a little horizontally to the next spot, and the next, etc.

Graston Technique®

The **Graston Technique**® is a patented form of soft tissue massage treatment that enables therapists to break down scar tissue and fascial restrictions using specially designed stainless steel instruments.

The concept of cross fiber massage has been around for some time. The new Graston Technique® uses specially designed instruments along with a new treatment protocol. The idea was originally developed by an athlete who suffered a debilitating knee injury while water skiing and was dissatisfied with his rehabilitation progress.

The Graston Technique® is based on six stainless steel instruments. Their shapes mold to the contours of the body and because metal instruments do not compress like the tips of fingers it allows deeper restrictions to be accessed and treated. The tools also save the therapist's hands. Standard treatment protocol includes warm-up exercises followed by Graston Technique® treatment which is then followed by stretching, strengthening and ice.

The first outpatient clinic to feature this process was opened in 1994 and today the Graston Technique® is used by a wide variety of therapists including chiropractors, athletic trainers, massage therapists and others.

`www.grastontechnique.com`

Indian Head Massage

Indian men and women have practiced a type of massage based on the Ayurvedic healing system for thousands of years to stimulate circulation and relieve tension. It's believed that when the scalp is loose blood flows more freely to feed the hair root in order to prevent hair loss. There are many different techniques but Narenda Mehta developed the **Champissage** style in the 1970s while in London studying to become a physiotherapist. His massage technique involves the head but also the neck, shoulders and back for a more thorough procedure.

`http://www.champissageinternational.com/`

Lomilomi Massage

Lomilomi is an ancient form of healing art from Hawaii. Legends say that students were said to study for more than 20 years and received their final instructions from their master on his death bed. There are many different styles of Lomilomi, usually based on where it was developed.

Muscle Energy Technique (MET)

Dr. Fred Mitchell, Sr. developed this process in the early 1960s as a comprehensive manual therapy system but today it is almost an umbrella term for a wide range of muscle relaxation or stretching techniques. Two fundamentals of this process are reciprocal inhibition (RI) and post-isometric relaxation (PIR). RI is the response when the therapist uses a client's muscle to stretch the opposing muscle. PIR is the relaxation response that follows when an isometric contraction is released. This form of massage can be used as a sports massage.

https://en.wikipedia.org/wiki/Muscle_energy_technique

Myofascial Release

Myofascial Release refers to the manual soft tissue manipulation techniques for stretching the fascia and releasing bonds between fascia and integument, muscles, and bones, with the goal of eliminating pain, increasing range of motion and balancing the body. See also *Myofacial Release*.

Myofascial Trigger Point Therapy or Trigger Point Therapy

 MTPT is a massage style to relieve pain and restricted motion. Trigger points are painful points in muscles which cause the surrounding fascia to shorten and become tight. Direct or indirect pressure on trigger points causes them to unwind. This technique is used by a wide range of therapists ranging from doctors to chiropractors to massage therapists. See also *Myofacial Release*

www.MyofascialTherapy.org

Neuromuscular Massage

Therapy usually used to treat muscle spasm. Using the fingers, knuckles or elbow alternating levels of pressure are used but remaining constant for ten to thirty seconds at each pressure level.

Petrissage Massage

Petrissage is one of the five basic strokes of a Swedish massage. It's a kneading movement performed with the whole palm or finger tips by wringing, skin rolling, compression and lifting vertically on the muscle tissue. Often useful for warming of tissue for deeper work it increases circulation, softens superficial fascia and decreases muscle tension.

Russian Clinical Massage

Russian Clinical Massage (RCM), also known as Russian Curative Massage is a cross-fiber technique with three distinct sections and 40+ movements. The first phase is slow for relaxation followed by the second fast and deep phase for therapeutic effect and then the slow third stage for relaxation and completion. The first massage school in Russia opened in the 17th century but the latest developments are claimed to reverse atrophy in muscles. The wide variety of techniques creates specific responses in the nervous system to speed up elimination of waste in the tissues, increase cell metabolism and recovery.

Shantala Massage

This type of ancient Indian technique is used to massage babies and children. It was introduced to the West by French obstetrician Dr. Frederique Leboyer and is described as a very simple technique. Its rhythmic movements help a child to relax, enhances their sense of security, sleep patterns and immune system.

www.ShantalaMassage.org

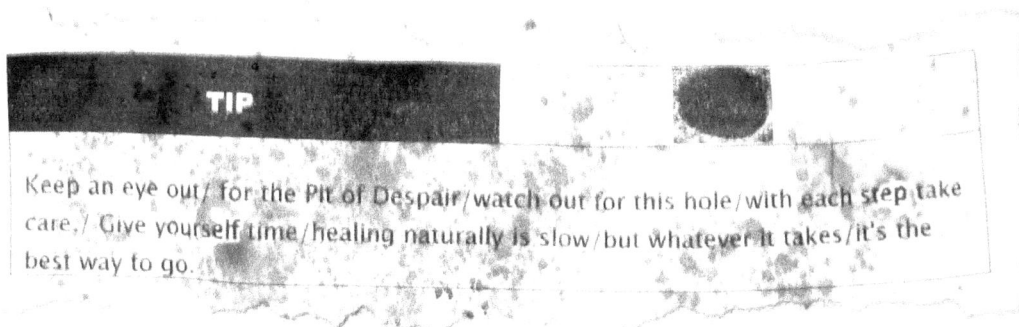

TIP

Keep an eye out/ for the Pit of Despair/watch out for this hole/with each step take care./ Give yourself time/healing naturally is slow/but whatever it takes/it's the best way to go.

Shiatsu

From the Japanese words meaning "finger" and "pressure" the fundamental concept of Shiatsu is diagnosis and therapy combined to correct imbalances in the body. The technique uses mainly the thumbs but also finger pressure or pressure from the palm of the hand to work all along the meridians of the body. The focus is on treating the entire meridian but effective points may also be used. Normally the client is fully clothed on a floor mat for this work. Tokujiro Namiloshi founded the Japan Shiatsu College in 1940 to standardize Shiatsu Therapy. It is used around the world for promoting health and aiding in the healing of illness. (see Asian Bodywork listing.)

There are different types of Shiatsu such as the *Five Element Shiatsu* method which uses four examinations to determine the best massage pattern to harmonize the body. It uses the paradigm of the five elements to modify or control patterns of disharmony.

Interactive Eclectic Shiatsu combines traditional Japanese Shiatsu techniques with Traditional Chinese Medicine and Western-style soft tissue manipulation methods. It also uses dietary and herbal features for a comprehensive treatment style.

Sports Massage

The purpose of Sports Massage is to prepare an athlete for peak performance, and afterwards to relieve fatigue, swelling and muscle tension to prevent injuries and promote flexibility. Complete workouts today include caring for the wear-and-tear that comes with exercise. Since each sport uses different muscles in different ways the massage therapist must customize the Sports Massage to each athlete. Normally this will involve a combination of massage techniques including Swedish and Shiatsu along with deep tissue, trigger point work and acupressure. Massages may be given before or after competition, or both in some cases.

Stone Massage

This method uses hot or cold stones, usually of basalt or marble, to massage the body. Stone sizes may vary from pebble to palm-sized and they may be placed directly on the skin or on a towel. They are usually placed on key energy points like energy meridians or chakras to improve energy flow. Depending on the technique the arrangement of stones may be in a straight line, dual lines similar to a cupping pattern in Traditional Chinese Medicine or other design. Using hot stones to give a deep massage creates a sensation of warmth while the heat relaxes the muscles and calms the nervous system. Hot stones also expand the blood vessels which help to push blood and waste through the body. It also allows for greater intensity than a regular massage.

When the client is suffering from any type of inflammation frozen or cooling stones are used to massage the body. In some cases both types of stones are used to stimulate the enlarging and then constricting of blood vessels for cleansing and healing.

Swedish Massage

The standard form of massage in the U.S. is the Swedish Massage which uses long, flowing strokes, often in the direction of the heart, to increase circulation and blood flow. There are six basic strokes which are applied with oil, cream or lotion to minimize the friction caused by a wider area of treatment. The types of strokes are effleurage, petrisage, friction, tapotement, compression and vibration. The approach was standardized by Dutch practitioner Johan Georg Mezger in the late 1800s.

USER COMMENTS:

- ◆ After doing four sessions last week, I felt better than I've felt in my adult life; more energized, joyous, and whole! It's hard to explain as I don't ever remember feeling this way, better circulation and so alive.

Thai massage

This style is based on the Ayurveda system which originated in India. Clients lie on a floor mat in loose, comfortable clothing while the practitioner puts the body into many yoga positions. The practitioner leans on the client using hands and forearms to apply firm, rhythmic pressure to the body. The two-hour process usually follows energy meridians called Sen Lines which are similar to TCM meridians.

Tui na

In Chinese the words mean "push-grasp" which describes this acupressure treatment used to bring the client's body back into balance. The massage therapist may brush, knead, press or rub the areas between each of the joints called the eight gates to get the chi energy moving again in the meridians and muscles. The therapist will use range of motion technique along with traction, massage and the stimulation of acupressure points based on the Eight Principles. It is a form of Chinese manipulative therapy and part of Traditional Chinese Medicine so it may be used with other elements of TCM.

MEDICAL RESEARCH

In a fascinating article in the ATLANTIC Magazine from November 2010 author David H. Freedman explains why so much of what medical researchers conclude in their studies is misleading, exaggerated, or flat-out wrong. The bigger question is why doctors continue to utilize these studies as part of their practice.

Dr. John Ioannidis has spent his career challenging his peers by exposing their bad science which doesn't make him very popular in medical circles. He's recognized as a meta-researcher, and he's become one of the world's foremost experts on the credibility of medical research. He charges that as much as 90 percent of the published medical information that doctors rely on is flawed. He worries that the field of medical research is so pervasively flawed, and so riddled with conflicts of interest, that it might be chronically resistant to change.

He first came upon the sorts of problems plaguing the field as a young physician-researcher in the early 1990s at Harvard. A new "evidence-based medicine" movement was just so he threw himself into it, working first with prominent researchers at Tufts University and then at Johns Hopkins University and the National Institutes of Health. In researching medical journals he was struck by how many findings of all types were refuted by later research.

Among his own findings he discovered that researchers headed into their studies wanting certain results—and they were getting them. In 2005, he unleashed two papers that challenged the foundations of medical research. He chose to publish one paper in the online journal *PLoS Medicine*, which is committed to running any methodologically sound article without regard to how "interesting" the results may be. He proved that 80 percent of non-randomized studies (by far the most common type) turn out to be wrong, as do 25 percent of supposedly gold-standard randomized trials, and as much as 10 percent of the platinum-standard large randomized trials. His second, similar, article was published in the *Journal of the American Medical Association Nature*, the grande dame of science journals, stated in a 2006 editorial: "Scientists understand that peer review per se provides only a minimal assurance of quality, and that the public conception of peer review as a stamp of authentication is far from the truth."

Ioannidis initially thought the medical community might come out fighting. Instead, it seemed relieved, as if it had been guiltily waiting for someone to blow the whistle, and eager to hear more. He says that "Doctors need to rely on instinct and judgment to make choices," he says. "But these choices should be as informed as possible by the evidence. And if the evidence isn't good, doctors should know that, too. And so should patients." He adds that "Science is a noble endeavor, but it's also a low-yield endeavor. I'm not sure that more than a very small percentage of medical research is ever likely to lead to major improvements in clinical outcomes and quality of life. We should be very comfortable with that fact."

`http://www.theatlantic.com/magazine/archive/2010/11/lies-damned-lies-and-medical-science/308269/`

MYOFASCIAL RELEASE

Myofascial Release is a technique of sustained pressure for eliminating pain and increasing the body's range of motion. Injuries, stress, trauma, overuse and poor posture can cause restriction to fascia. Myofascial release frees fascial restrictions, and allows the muscles to move efficiently. This is usually done by applying shear, compression or tension in various directions, or by skin rolling. There are two main schools of myofascial release: direct and indirect methods.

Dr. Janet Travell began using the term "Myofascial Trigger Point" in 1976, so a variation of the technique is known as **Myofascial Trigger Point Therapy**

The fascia system is a single network of coverings on muscles, bones and organs that runs from head to foot connecting every part of the body. Its normal healthy condition is relaxed with the ability to stretch and move. When muscles are injured, stressed or inflamed their fibers and the surrounding fascia become short and tight, a condition which can spread to other locations in the body restricting motion and causing discomfort.

Practitioners using the direct method or deep tissue work use their knuckles, elbows or tools with sufficient pressure to slowly sink into the constricted fascia to stretch the fibers, allowing the tissue to reorganize into a more flexible manner.

A more gentle approach using lighter pressure is called the indirect method. This employs a stretching motion to allow the fascia to release or unwind itself. This technique uses the body's natural ability for self correction which often produces increased blood flow to the area and warmth.

The John F. Barnes' Myofascial Release Approach seminars are one source for this type of specialized training. There are also seminars available to learn how to use this technique to treat yourself.

`www.myofascialrelease.com`

USER COMMENTS:

♦ My injury was three years old and I had spent over $30,000 when I arrived at the John F. Barnes Myofascial Release Treatment Center. It was my last resort. The program that I went through changed my life. After only seven days at the John F. Barnes Myofascial Release Treatment Center, I was able to turn my neck around in circles.

♦ Even though I was receiving good, traditional therapy, I continued to lose strength and functional mobility in my arms and shoulders. I was desperately discouraged and always in significant pain. Once I started receiving comprehensive therapy through the John F. Barnes Myofascial Release Treatment Center, I made more progress in two weeks than I had in the previous year. The therapists also helped me set up a home exercise program so I could continue to improve and have a more functional, pain free life.

NAMBUDRIPAD ALLERGY ELIMINATION TECHNIQUE (NAET)

The **Nambudripad Allergy Elimination Technique** (NAET) was developed by Dr. Devi S. Nambudripad, M.D., D.C., Lac, PhD. (Acu.) in 1983. As a California acupuncturist, chiropractor and kinesiologist she created the natural, drugless, non-invasive process to deal with allergies and their health consequences.

NAET eliminates allergies using a combination of muscle testing, selective energy balancing using acupuncture or acupressure, nutrition, chiropractic techniques and traditional medicine. Neuromuscular Sensitivity Testing (NST) uses straight arm kinesiology techniques to evaluate the relative strength and weakness of the body's reaction to different substances. Following diagnosis one allergen is treated at a time in a specific sequence. In many cases a single treatment may successfully treat an allergen. An average person may have 15-20 food and environmental allergens which would require 15-20 office visits.

Training and certification in the technique is done by Dr. Nambudripad in basic and advanced seminars. Many NAET practitioners are chiropractors or acupuncturists.

`www.naet.com`

USER COMMENTS:

♦ I almost lost my life. I was suffering from Crohn's disease. In and out of the hospital—and as every Crohn's patient discovers—treatment (other than surgical interventions), becomes large doses of prednisone (steroids) or other immuno-suppressant drugs. NAET saved my life, treatments addressed the CAUSE of Crohn's disease. My ongoing struggle to lower the dosage of prednisone was frustrated at 35 mg. Then, after just a few treatments of NAET, to handle the vicious food allergies, I was able to drop the dose from 35 mg to 10 mg WITH NO ADVERSE AFFECTS. There were no excessive symptoms of bleeding or starvation or relapse of the disease.

♦ Ten months ago, I injured my shoulder when I was lifting with my trainer. Over the course of the following nine months, I tried a multitude of things to heal my shoulder. Not only did the above endeavors fail, my shoulder continued to have less and less mobility. After going through the first five NAET treatments, you tested me for acrylic nails. WOW! I tested a definite yes for the nails causing my shoulder impingement! Little did I expect such amazing results so quickly after my acrylic treatment. Within two weeks I had fifty percent mobility in my shoulder. Within four weeks I am at ninety-five percent improved. I am sure that last five percent will soon improve with a few laser treatments you have planned. My trainer was in amazement at the fast improvement. Obviously, NAET works!

♦ From my experience, doctors are rushed and unable to explain things properly. They tend to offer medication rather than finding out the real source of 'why' you are in the state that you are in. There are a lot of answers out there, but that it's always going to be up to us to sift through it all and find what works best. In my search of alternative therapies and treatments, I discovered a NAET practitioner. She has been a huge help and inspiration to me along the way and has already cleared me of a few of the many allergies that I have.

♦ One of my most stubborn allergies to date has been an allergy to cats. Normally I couldn't spend more than 5 minutes near a cat before starting to experience wheezing, shortness of breath, and just basically felt miserable. The symptoms lasted far after leaving where the cats were and honestly it was a huge inconvenience in my life. After two treatments I can proudly state that I'm officially cleared of the cat allergy. Wow... what a blessing this has been!

TIP

To follow your path/you will always find/walking in sunshine/helps all mankind.

NAPRAPATHY

Naprapathy was introduced in the U.S. by Dr. Oakley Smith in 1907 as a treatment process for evaluating and healing damaged connective tissues. The term comes from the Czech word "naprapravit" meaning "to connect" and the Greek word "pathos" for "suffering". This treatment technique for structural imbalances deals with sources of pain which often begin in the spine and spread throughout the body causing locomotor disorders. His discovery of this therapy was the result of his own lifelong search for better health which had already tried chiropractic care and osteopathy. He found this new system used bones as levers with a gentle motion and was a different type of therapy.

Poor posture, trauma from sports injuries or whiplash, and even general wear can be the cause of the imbalances which cause the deterioration of the suppleness in connective tissues like ligaments. Such inelastic tissues produce stiffness which can progress to cause pinched nerves, contributing to health problems like arthritis, carpal tunnel syndrome, Temporomandibular Joint (TMJ) Syndrome and other aches and pains.

The primary method of treatment by Doctors of Naprapathy (DN) is manipulation of the spine focusing on the underlying ligaments along with the joints and soft tissues. Practitioners of Naprapathy, or Naprapaths, can also use ultrasound, electrical pain relief treatments along with heat and cold therapies and even lasers. To assist treatments they may also use back braces, neckbands, taping and various types of joint supports along with posture and dietary counseling. Patients learn to appreciate their responsibility for their own health with a goal of decreasing dependence on therapy.

The National College of Naprapathic Medicine in Chicago is the original school of Naprapathy and it remains the only one offering programs to receive a DN or Doctor of Naprapathy degree. Naprapaths are licensed in Illinois and New Mexico, regulated in Ohio and may practice in other states that offer freedom of access statutes.

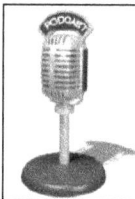

> Dr. Wayne Cichowicz is the Academic Dean of the National College of Naprapathic Medicine in Chicago, the only school of Naprapathy in America. We had a delightful conversation about this 100-year-old therapy brought from Europe by Dr. Oakley Smith.

http://napmed.edu, http://www.naprapathy.org

NATUROPATHY

Naturopathy or naturopathic medicine is a therapy to help the body's ability to heal by employing a variety of techniques. It may use acupuncture, aromatherapy, counseling, hydrotherapy, manual therapy and other techniques. Believing in the healing power of nature, this process recognizes that stressful lifestyles, poor diet and other factors can weaken a person, allowing bacteria and viruses to become a problem in the body. It also focuses on preventing health problems by promoting health maintenance by lifestyle changes. This type of medicine looks at the whole person instead of just specific symptoms or health issues. According to the 2007 federal survey 0.3% of respondents had used Naturopathy in the previous 12 months.

There are two schools of naturopathy today, naturopathic physicians who may use drugs and minor surgery and naturopaths who adhere to a completely natural and holistic process using the body's natural healing ability. Both treat patients as whole beings with a preference for natural therapies like foods and herbs.

Benedict Lust brought natural health practices like hydrotherapy to America from Germany and opened the first School of Naturopathy in New York in 1905. The concept grew in popularity and for a time was conventional medicine before the shift to artificial drugs and then nearly became extinct before gradually being rediscovered by the public in the 1950s.

Today, naturopathic physicians are licensed in 16 states. To become a licensed physician they must have a Doctor of Naturopathic Medicine (N.D. or N.M.D.) or Doctor of Naturopathy degree from an accredited institution and pass the required licensing board exams. Please be aware that a D.N.M. or Doctor of Natural Medicine degree does not qualify to be licensed as a naturopathic physician and carries no regulatory status in this country.

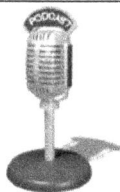

Dr. Lise Alschuler, the President of the American Association of Naturopathic Physicians talked with me about how this therapy bridges natural and conventional medicine. Dr. Alschuler is Board certified in naturopathic oncology and has been in practice for 14 years.

`www.naturopathic.org, www.anma.com`

NETWORK SPINAL ANALYSIS™ CARE (NSA)

Network Spinal Analysis™ Care is a networking of different chiropractic techniques using gentle, specific touches in a consistent sequence to produce healing waves of relaxation. Developed in 1982 by New York chiropractor Dr. Donald Epstein the process enables chiropractors to release large amounts of spinal tension from patients.

By using light touch to the spine the patient's body learns to release patterns of tension, resulting in even deeper tensions being released. The finger or light hand contact is applied to specific access points along the neck and lower spine called spinal gateways which produces two waves of healing. The first is a breathing wave which releases immediate tension throughout the body to relax the patient. The second wave is a body-mind wave which corresponds to the relaxing motion of the spine.

The spine is a string of bones in our back sitting one on top of the other with pads called discs in between each one. Each vertebra has a hole, the spinal canal, where the spinal cord runs from the base of your brain to your tail bone. The connective tissues which attach this whole system to the body respond to all of the stresses and tensions of your life which impacts the functioning of your body. Using NSA to release tension and retrain the body how to release tension, patients become more peaceful and at ease with their life which improves healing capacity and wellness.

Effective Spring 2012, the Association for Network Care was dissolved as an organization. Their old website now forwards to:

`www.reorganizational.org`

USER COMMENTS:

♦ As a complete non-believer who'd never even gone to a chiropractor you can imagine how bad the pain in my neck was to get me to try NSA, but a good friend said it was very effective even if it was a little strange. She said it was more like touching than a regular chiropractic adjustment. He talked with me before the first session to get my medical history and then had me lay down on the massage table. He did some gentle touch around my back and then did this motion with his thumb at the bottom of my spine. Afterwards he stepped away for a few minutes so he could watch my breathing to see the blockages and then he worked on the other side of my back. He warned me that I might feel a little light headed and to get up slowly, and he was right.

♦ My co-workers noticed a major change in my attitude after just the first session although it took several more visits to really deal with the stress. Things just didn't bother me the same way and I deal with problems more effectively.

♦ Some sessions I'd cry and other sessions I'd laugh but the therapist said it was all very normal and natural, I was simply releasing a lot of locked up emotions which were causing me stress. Best of all the neck pain completely disappeared and I've found a greater sense of calm and peace.

NEUROMODULATION TECHNIQUE (NMT)

The **NeuroModulation Technique** (NMT) or the **Feinberg Technique** is based on muscle testing (Applied Kinesiology) to access the body's control mechanisms to restore its ability to heal. It was developed in 2002 by Dr. Leslie S. Feinberg as the result of 20 years of energetic therapy research and his chiropractic experience, combining Western science with energy medicine.

The process uses active muscle testing along with passive muscle testing, which is observing the response by the shortening or lengthening of a leg or arm. The process sequence first accesses the body's system to measure the errors causing the problem and finally to correct the situation by restoring the control system to normal operation.

"It can be hard to figure out just which symptoms are for what problem."
- Karen

Normally the patient is seated on a backless swivel chair so the practitioner can muscle test and treat easily. After each step the patient uses patterned breathing while the practitioner uses a special FDA approved device to stimulate vertebra with gentle taps. There may be variations of technique by practitioners depending on the situation.

Following an initial examination a practitioner will report the findings and discuss a reasonable schedule for improvement. Frequently it will take six to twelve sessions to reach the desired treatment milestones but since every individual and condition are unique, the results can vary.

www.NeuroModulationTechnique.com

NEW BIOLOGY or Epigenetics

The science of **epigenetics** is the study of molecular mechanisms used by the environment to control gene activity. This is a paradigm shift about the functioning of the human body, a reversal in the perspective of traditional medicine.

The field is commonly referred to as the **New Biology** and research scientist Bruce Lipton, Ph.D. is considered one of its most popular spokesmen. His research on cloned stem cells revealed that genes themselves did not control life, but that our biology and behavior are primarily determined by our perceptions of the world. In other words our thoughts, feelings and beliefs control the functions of our genes. What was once considered magic or metaphysical is today's science.

Cellular and molecular biology research during the last decade like the Human Genome Project is proving to be a catalyst for revolution in conventional medical science. It has shown that cell behavior and genetic expression are directly influenced by information derived from the environment, including energy. Epigenetics means over and above genetics. Rather than a bottom-up belief where genes within the cell control life, the new top-down philosophy has the nervous system, with its perceptions, attitudes and beliefs, controlling genes. (*also see* **Psychoneuroimmunology**.) However current biology textbooks and mass media continue to promote outdated concepts perpetuating a victim mentality.

One area demonstrating how thoughts affect human biology is called **neuroplasticity**. With assistance from the Dalai Lama, researchers have begun to discover how years of meditation can change the actual functioning of the brain in an enduring manner.

Dr. Lipton has been a teacher and/or researcher at many outstanding institutions, including The University of Virginia, The University of Wisconsin's School of Medicine, Stanford University's School of Medicine, The University of Puerto Rico's School of Medicine and Penn State University. His ground-breaking book, *The Biology of Belief*, was selected as the Best Science Book in the Best Books 2006 Awards.

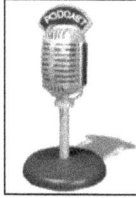

> Dr. Lipton's breakthrough studies on the cell membrane revealed that the outer layer of the cell was the equivalent of a brain which led to the new science of Epigenetics and the New Biology. Dr. Lipton is an international authority on bridging science and spirit.

www.brucelipton.com

NUTRITION

There are literally hundreds of books available about diets and supplements so I've chosen to skip this topic. The main reason is that I'm just as confused as everyone else. There are diets from Atkins to Zone and everything in between, each with its own philosophy and supporting research. While I heartily agree that proper nutrition is a vital part of every health program I'm leaving this research to you.

The field of supplements is even more confusing. There are books devoted strictly to supplements that are several inches thick. Again, you'll have to figure this one out on your own but I'll at least give you a place to start:

www.dietary-supplements.info.nih.gov/,
www.nutrition.gov, www.nutrition.org or www.eatright.org

ORNISH PROGRAM

The **Ornish Program** can stop and even reverse heart disease without drugs or surgery. His bestselling book *Dr. Dean Ornish's Program For Reversing Heart Disease* was first published in 1990 presenting scientific evidence on the success of his 4-step program. In it Dr. Eugene Braunwald, the chief of medicine at Harvard Medical School, was quoted on his reaction after he watched the PBS special on The Ornish Program. Dr. Braunwald said "Dr. Ornish's study is scientifically valid but it'll never play in Peoria." This statement reflects the attitude of many in the mainstream medical community which is why this program is included as a complimentary or alternative therapy. However Medicare approved it in 2008 as the first lifestyle therapy in Medicare history so attitudes are slowly changing.

Dr. Ornish began to question the fundamental premise of heart therapy at the very beginning of his medical career. He asked what would be the difference if patients changed the underlying cause of their heart problems instead of merely treating the symptoms with drugs and surgery. While insurance companies would gladly pay $50,000 for a heart by-pass operation or $5,000 to implant a stent to open an artery they couldn't see the benefit in spending a dime on prevention. This short-sighted approach has improved slightly but the insurance industry still has not sufficiently embraced the concepts of prevention.

The first step Dr. Ornish recommends is to quit smoking. For anyone with heart problems this step is abundantly clear in this day and age and does not require further explanation.

The special diet he recommends is very restrictive because that is what it takes to reverse heart disease. Losing weight can be done simply by eating less fat and fewer simple carbohydrates but reversing heart disease requires a radical change in diet to a vegetarian program balanced for proper nutrition.

Emotional stress is a key factor in this program because stress makes arteries constrict and blood clot faster which can lead to a heart attack. Stress management in the program involves yoga stretching, relaxation breathing techniques, meditation and guided imagery along with support groups. Sharing and connecting with other people can have a profoundly beneficial effect on stress.

The last part of the program is an extension of the emotional factor involving love and intimacy. Studies have shown that those who are lonely and depressed are more likely to get sick than those who have a strong family connections, deep personal relationships and active participation in their community.

Dr. Ornish asks heart patients a simple question: How much do you want to live? If they are willing to make all of the necessary changes to their lives then their heart disease can be reversed.

Based on the success of his health program Dr. Ornish's newest book and program is called *The Spectrum*. This is about how to personalize a way of eating and a way of living based on your own health goals and preferences based on a joy of living instead of a fear of dying. Built on the concepts of his original work each personalized plan contains 3 components: Nutrition, Stress Management, and Exercise.

It's interesting to note that the 2007 federal survey chose only to survey the "Ornish Diet" instead of listing it as a lifestyle therapy. Only 77 people responded so it had a 0.0% response rate, possibly because of the poor classification.

`www.pmri.org/spectrum/`

USER COMMENTS:

♦ I was scared. Lying in bed in the still of the night my heart didn't sound like it had for the previous 55 years of my life. The beat was irregular, it not only sounded funny, it also felt strange. Weeks of tests labeled the condition an electrical problem, not a blockage but I wasn't going to take any chances with my life. Diet, exercise and any other changes that I had to make got made ... quickly. Fear is a powerful motivator for change!

♦ The Ornish diet program is a tough change for a meat-and-potatoes guy. I probably had more vegetables in the first month on the program than I've had in the last year (or more)! Some of the recipes weren't too bad, they were modifications of foods I was already used to, but some were pretty strange.

♦ Most of us never find the time to exercise but when your life depends on it, it's amazing how fast it becomes the #1 priority! Have to admit I was in pretty sad shape when I started but months into the program the results are starting to show. Meditation took some real dedication in the beginning but you can get used to it pretty quickly.

♦ All in all, it's clear the program really does work. In the first month my triglycerides dropped by 1/3 and my total cholesterol level dropped into the normal range for the first time in my life. I'm happier, healthier and have more joy in my life than ever before so now I'm a walking testimonial for The Ornish Program.

ORTHOMOLECULAR MEDICINE

The term "orthomolecular" was created by two-time Nobel Prize winner and molecular biologist, Linus Pauling, Ph.D at the end of the 1960s. The term "orthomolecular" comes from "ortho", Greek for "correct" or "right," and "molecule" so it can be defined as the "right molecule." It focuses on the use of naturally occurring substances in maintaining health and treating disease. Although *UnBreak Your Health* doesn't include information on diets and supplements this general listing on **Orthomolecular Medicine** is included because the field also uses several therapies that are listed here including: chelation therapy; hydrotherapy; phototherapy; electrotherapy; light therapy; solar therapy; acupuncture; massage; biofeedback; hypnotherapy and other therapies.

The importance of nutrition to health goes back more than 2,500 years ago to Hippocrates and even to ancient Egypt. Dr. James Lind, a physician in the British navy, was the first person to show a direct link between disease and diet in 1757 when he discovered that sailors on long voyages without rations containing citrus fruits developed scurvy. The term "limeys" refers to the fact British sailors were supplied with lemons and limes afterwards so they could sail around the world without the disease caused by vitamin C deficiency.

Orthomolecular Medicine is built on the scientific foundations of nutrition, biochemistry and clinical nutrition. While practitioners do not deny the value of pharmaceutical drugs they recognize their limitations and their potential for toxicity and prefer instead to use nutrition as the first and primary course of treatment. Another key feature is the concept of biochemical individuality. Basic nutrition guidelines from government agencies are ineffective due to the metabolism variations and dietary necessities within each individual. Practitioners promote environmental medicine with their belief that pollution and food adulteration are a fact of life in the modern world and therefore a medical priority.

www.orthomed.org, www.orthomolecular.org

OSTEOPATHIC MEDICINE

Osteopathic Medicine or Osteopathy is a holistic approach to healthcare recognizing the unity of all body parts and the body's ability to heal itself. A U.S. Army doctor, Andrew Taylor Still, M.D., founded Osteopathy in 1874. In this philosophy of health, a human being is more than simply the sum of its body parts. Osteopathy is considered a separate but equal branch of medical care in this country having become integrated with mainstream medicine in 1969. However, outside the U.S., where it has remained essentially a drug free system based on manipulative techniques, it is still considered a complementary process.

Doctors of Osteopathy, or D.O.s, receive full medical training of four years of medical school, three to six years of internship or residency and additional training just like mainstream or allopathic physicians. D.O.s receive extra training in the musculoskeletal system, the relationship between the muscles, bones and nerves, so they better understand how a problem in one part of the body can impact other areas.

D.O.s are trained to use their hands to help diagnose and treat injury and illness using **osteopathic manipulative treatment** or OMT. This involves moving the muscles and joints with stretching, resistance and the gentle use of pressure to properly align the body. However they also recognize that sometimes medication and surgery may be required therapy.

These are the eight generally accepted principles of osteopathy including concepts like "the body is a unit" and "structure and function are interrelated". They appreciate how body fluids are essential to health and that nerves play a vital role in the motion of fluids. The body can heal itself but maintaining health today is a constant struggle against stress, environmental toxins and other challenges. They believe in a holistic approach to health to prevent illness.

After enduring the horrors of the Civil War battlefield and then the loss of his wife and children from disease, Dr. Still lost his faith in the standard medicine of the day. Conventional medicine at that time was using mercury as medicine. He began researching and testing other methods of healing and in 1892 founded the American School of Osteopathy in Kirksville, Missouri as the first medical school of its kind in the world. His methods attracted a great deal of unpleasant attention at the time and Kirksville was one of the few places that allowed him to practice. Today it's called Andrew Taylor Still University, Kirksville College of Osteopathic Medicine. Although Missouri was willing to grant him a charter for awarding medical doctor degrees, he was so unhappy with the field that he chose to issue his own D.O. degree.

Both Doctors of Osteopathy and Medical Doctors must pass comparable examinations to obtain state licenses to practice medicine and work in fully accredited and licensed healthcare facilities.

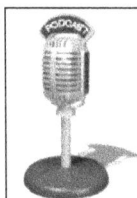

Dr. Philip Slocum, Dean of the Kirksville College of Osteopathic Medicine (KCOM) at A.T. Still University was my very first podcast program interview. Our conversation was on the history of the uniquely American medical system of Osteopathy, the benefits it offers patients today and how it helps the body heal naturally.

www.osteopathic.org, www.atsu.edu/kcom/

OZONE THERAPY

Ozone Therapy is a healing treatment that introduces ozone into the body. All 30 or so **oxygen therapies,** including ozone therapy, flood the body with single atoms (oxygen is O^2 and ozone is O^3). By putting large quantities of ozone into the body the single oxygen molecule that is unattached circulates freely to attack a wide range of illness and disease. It is considered to be anti-viral, anti-bacterial, anti-fungal because these organisms cannot live in an oxygen-rich environment. It is also said to have antioxidant stimulating capabilities.

This process normally uses an oxygen generator connected with an ozone generator to produce precisely controlled amounts of ozone. It may be introduced into the body in a variety of ways including:

1) Ingestion: drinking water or consuming olive oil that has been infused with ozone.
2) Rectal Insufflation: introducing ozone through the colon.
3) Vaginal Insufflation: introducing ozone into the female body.
4) Insertion in the Ear: placing the tube directly into the ear.
5) Transdermal (or through the skin): using a variety of methods including a baths, body suit, wraps or bagging, and other techniques.
6) Injection: placing ozone directly into the body in specially-prepared fluids, sometimes directly into a tumor site.
7) Inhalation: breathing in ozone directly, often using a sauna.

As an example, rectal insufflation is done by inserting the delivery tube directly into the colon so that humidified ozone can be absorbed directly into the bloodstream. If the large intestine is lined with debris the absorption rate is decreased. Treatments vary but often the first week's therapy uses a 30-second session for one to three days.

In America the first use of ozone therapy was by Dr. John H. Kellogg at his Battle Creek, Michigan sanitarium using ozone steam saunas in 1880. Since that time ozone therapy has been recognized in several countries around the world as an effective healing therapy.

Two of the most popular books are *Oxygen Therapies: A New Way of Approaching Disease* by Ed McCabe (1988) and his latest work *Flood Your Body With Oxygen* (2002).

The International Association for Oxygen Therapy was founded in 1972 to promote the use of ozone and other oxygen therapies. In the U.S. ozone therapy is usually taught privately or in naturopathic schools so it is wise to check the training and qualifications along with state regulations before beginning this type of therapy.

`www.ozoneuniversity.com`

USER COMMENTS:

♦ I cured my asthma with the attachment where you breathe the ozone through olive oil. My asthma had been so bad that I couldn't even lie down when I slept and my MD had me on massive doses of steroids (which I stopped to do this therapy). It took five months, but I have remained asthma free with only occasional maintenance touch ups. An unexpected benefit to the treatment was that my eyesight improved.

PILATES

Pilates is a physical education program developed by Joseph Hubertus Pilates in the early part of the twentieth century. It is a set of principles and full-body, sequential exercises which works the whole body in balance, coordinating the upper and lower parts of the body with its center or core.

Born in Germany in 1880 Pilates was a frail child but grew up to become an accomplished athlete, gymnast and boxer. During World War I he was held in detention camps in England where he became a nurse and devised exercises for immobilized patients. He opened the first Pilates Studio in New York City in 1926. His first book was *Your Health* published in 1932 which was followed by *Return To Life Through Contrology* in 1945.

Originally called **Contrology** it focuses on the core postural muscles which help keep the body balanced and provide support for the spine. Pilates exercises teach awareness of breath and alignment of the spine. Programs are uniquely tailored to each individual which is why it can be used to treat health problems. It is very popular with dancers and performers because it builds strength and flexibility without bulk. It became known as the Pilates Method after the death of Joseph Pilates in 1967.

Pilates exercises demand complete, intense focus because they teach body awareness. The Pilates Method is a series of precision movements that engage both body and mind. The eight original principles of Pilates are: Concentration; Control; Centering; Flow; Precision; Breath; Relaxation and Stamina. The initial Pilates program contained 34 floor exercises but Joseph Pilates also invented several pieces of equipment with their own series of exercises. He developed the concept of the first one while serving in a detention camp in England. Using the springs from his bed he created the forerunner of the Reformer apparatus although some sources claim it was the Cadillac device.

"As we get older it gets harder to keep good health, things just seem to wear out."
- Karen

There are a variety of Pilates certifications available today so consumers are cautioned to research the training of their instructor because it is key to their ability to customize the program. Two of the main Pilates organizations today are the United States Pilates Association and the Pilates Method Alliance.

`www.unitedstatespilatesassociation.com, www.pilatesmethodalliance.org`

PLACEBO EFFECT

The **Placebo Effect** comes from the Latin phrase "I shall please" and it is used to describe the body's ability to heal itself. This completely natural type of healing should be the goal of every person since this type of healing has no side effects and no toxic chemicals. One of the first research reports on the process was *The Powerful Placebo* (1955) and it concluded that an average of 32% of patients responded to the placebo.

Research today with the newest technology is unlocking many of the secrets of the placebo effect but it's also creating even more questions about this powerful human ability. Researchers in Italy have discovered that there isn't one placebo effect but many different types. Researchers in the U.S. have found that the process isn't simply a psychological phenomenon as originally thought but is a real, physical response to belief and expectation. Neuroscientist Helen Mayberg discovered in 2002 that inert pills (placebos) work the same way on brains of depressed people as antidepressants. Activity in the seat of higher thought, the frontal cortex, increased while activity in the area for emotions, the limbic regions, decreased.

Anatomy of Hope (2003) by Harvard Medical School physician Jerome Groopman, M.D. says that "A change of mind-set can alter neurochemistry both in a laboratory setting and in the clinic." Dr. Groopman experienced the power of the placebo effect releasing the brain's endorphins and enkephlins to relieve his own back pain.

The Allen Brain Atlas, founded by Microsoft co-founder Paul Allen, was completed in 2006. The project researched where each gene was activated in a mouse's brain because of its many similarities to human brains. They discovered that 80% of the 21,000 genes in a mouse body were activated in the brain, more than anyone expected. This is a possible indication of the scope of the mind-body connection and the power of the placebo effect. This may also be a window into the function of epigenetics (*see New Biology*).

Medically inactive pills, often called sugar pills, are used to simulate real medications during testing of new medications to determine if they're more effective than the placebo effect. If the new product can't produce positive results higher than the placebo then it will not be approved by the Food and Drug Administration (FDA). The pharmaceutical industry has successfully tainted the term "placebo effect" with a very negative connotation because to them it's a real problem with financial consequences. However it should be remembered that the placebo effect is a powerful healing process. Because it can't be patented and sold for a profit this all-natural healing capacity has a negative effect on the modern drug industry but a very positive effect on patients.

Unfortunately for the drug industry the rate of positive responses to placebos have improved over the years as a result of better test design and the use of so-called active placebos which provide a detectable response unrelated to the problem. The better the placebo response the more difficult it is for new drugs to demonstrate effectiveness.

`www.pbs.org/wgbh/pages/frontline/shows/altmed/snake/placebo.html`

RAINDROP TECHNIQUE

The Raindrop Technique is a combination of aromatherapy, massage and reflexology designed to bring the body into structural and electrical alignment. The 8-step process was developed by Don Gary Young, N.D. and introduced in his book *Raindrop Technique* (2003).

The process was inspired by the healing practices of the Lakota Indians. It uses aromatic essential oils dropped like rain from a height of about six inches above the back and massaged into the back muscles along the vertebrae. Oils are also used to treat special locations on the feet in a modified form of reflexology. The process is reported to be particularly effective for abnormalities in the spine.

Young is also the founder of the Young Living Essential Oils company.

`www.younglivingworld.com/resources/raindrop_main.asp`

USER COMMENTS:

♦ I have a daughter who struggled with a lot of achiness due to undiagnosed Lyme Disease for three years. Her main struggles were muscle aches and overall fatigue. I started using the Raindrop Technique® as described in the Essential Oils Desk Reference. Within ten minutes of using it, I have a symptom-free, energetic ten-year-old again.

♦ I hurt my back in November 2004. I was in severe pain all day every day for months; sometimes it was excruciating. In June 2005, I started doing yoga, which helped, but I still felt bad pain. Then in August, I began having Raindrop Technique® done on me. Each time I have a treatment with the oils, I make a major leap forward—less pain and more mobility. By October I had a pain-free week. It is a real boon to be getting my life back. I am on the mend and expect to be completely well soon.

RELOX™ PROCEDURE

The **Relox**™ procedure was created to help stroke victims recover function. The process combines nutrition and oxygen for synergy of the components. Nutritional therapy involves taking vitamins and minerals both orally and intravenously. At the same time patients are receiving oxygen by standard face mask technique.

In many cases **Hyperbaric Oxygen Therapy** *(see listing)* is also used as part of the therapy to magnify the effectiveness of the Relox™ procedure. This is the application of pure oxygen at higher than normal pressures. HBOT chambers were originally designed to help deep sea divers recover from a condition known as "the bends" resulting from insufficient decompression. Today the technique is used for a variety of conditions involving circulation problems.

The process was developed by Bruce Rind, M.D., a board certified anesthesiologist with both traditional and alternative training, working in the Washington, D.C. area.

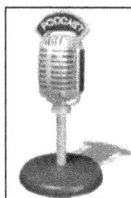

Dr. Bruce Rind is the creator of the Relox Procedure for healing stroke and other brain injuries. His unique combination of training in anesthesiology, nutrition and osteopathy combined to meet the needs of his patients in an effective new procedure.

www.drrind.com

USER COMMENTS:

♦ Seven years ago, I injured my ankle. The pain and swelling were constant. I could barely walk. My orthopedist recommended fusing the bones, which he said would cause me to lose all ankle/foot motion. There was no guarantee the pain or swelling would go away. I decided to find an alternative to that approach. Dr. Rind treated my ankle with prolotherapy. After five treatments, all the pain and swelling were gone. Since then, I hike several miles daily on my farm. The pain has not returned since.

♦ I was in a near fatal car accident in 1997. I was in a coma for one month. When I came out of it, I couldn't move, speak or remember anyone I knew from before. After a few months my memory started to return and I began a rehabilitation program for speech and walking. Rehab lasted nine months. My speech was slurred, walking was difficult and I could walk ten feet per minute.

I remained this way until Relox therapy. Within one hour of the first treatment, my speech, walking, balance and short term memory all had visibly and dramatically improved. At first I thought I was dreaming. By the next day I realized that my life had changed in a very positive way. I received one more treatment which included osteopathic adjustment. After that treatment my walking improved noticeably.

ROLFING®

Rolfing® Structural Integration was created in the 1950s by Dr. Ida Pauline Rolf as a holistic system of soft tissue manipulation and movement education. It's a unique blend of function and structure enabling the body to work in proper alignment with gravity.

In 1920 Ida Rolf received her Ph.D. in biochemistry. As a result of her own and others' health issues she researched the problems of bones, muscles and movement. One of her popular quotes is "Some individuals may perceive their losing fight with gravity as a sharp pain in their back, others as the unflattering contour of their body, others as constant fatigue...They are off balance. They are at war with gravity."

"This one seems to have helped, I move with less pain now."
- Karen

Her study of Hatha Yoga influenced the development of Rolfing. She recognized that bodies which are properly aligned and functioning with gravity have less stress and pain with more energy, improved posture and body awareness. The legs are aligned to the hips, shoulders and rib cage with the body positioned correctly over the feet so that all of the joints are integrated to each other.

Rolfing begins with the Ten Series, a basic sequence of ten one-hour sessions with the patient lying down on a massage table. At times the client will be asked to walk back and forth to evaluate progress. Each session has a specific goal in the sequence. While the client is guided through each movement the Rolfer manipulates the fascia to restore it to its original length applying slow-moving pressure with their knuckles, thumbs, fingers, elbows and even knees. Working with the deep myofascial structures to separate layers and align muscles the process acquired a reputation for being painful in the 1960s. Today most Rolfers work closely with clients for comfort and effectiveness.

After the initial sessions many clients choose a tune-up series. There is also an Advanced Series of five sessions available. Today, many Rolfers also offer movement training to compliment the structural integration.

In 1989, a group of dedicated followers started the Guild for Structural Integration to maintain Ida Rolf's traditional work and "the Recipe". This group of educators and practitioners has its own training programs and certification standards for GSI practitioners.

The Rolf Institute of Structural Integration (RISI) is another organization that trains and certifies Rolfers and Rolf Movement Practitioners around the world. Practitioners in the U.S. must be licensed as massage therapists, please check your state agencies for requirements.

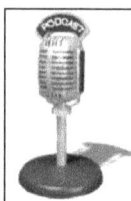

> Rolf Structural Integration is a type of body therapy developed by Dr. Ida Rolf. Although Ida Rolf and Moshe Feldenkrais were contemporaries in California and friends, their therapies were quite different. In this interview with Susan Melchoir, the School Director at the Rolf Guild in Boulder, Colorado, you'll learn about the differences in the techniques.

www.rolf.org or www.rolfguild.org

USER COMMENTS:

♦ Rolfing is about the good hurt, but after being all bent over and out of place, anything seems like an improvement. Actually, it IS a big improvement. Working with a 'gentle Rolfer' it didn't seem like there was a lot of movement going on, but man did it feel like it the next day. Walking back and forth over and over felt like different people were doing the walking. After all of the Ten Series sessions it's amazing how grounded you feel, also taller, stronger and more coordinated. There is just a grace and flow after everything has been put back together again. I will admit that additional 'tune-up' sessions were needed but after more than 50 years of gravity it wasn't a big surprise.

♦ I am sold on Rolfing because I get to do all the sports I want to even though I don't have a perfect back. Rolfing does not correct the inherent changes in my back, but it allows me to continue to do rigorous activities and makes me more aware of my body and helps with the pain, discomfort and stiffness. Rolfing gives me pain relief and keeps me symmetric so I can count on my body more.

♦ Massage offers immediate relief, but it's not lasting. Muscles endure repetitive strain. A simple injury with a suitcase can develop into a shoulder cramp, the muscle shortens from strain. Rolfing returns you to your optimum and balances your body. Chiropractic is like massage, it offers temporary relief, but you have to keep going back, the underlying problem is still there. Rolfing straightens out the underlying problem. It helps me with downhill and cross-country skiing, and bicycling which require balance. Having the body in balance supports my athletic interests."

TAI CHI or Tai Chi Chuan or T'ai Chi Ch'üan or Taijiquan

Tai Chi is a soft style, or relaxed form, of the martial arts. It is based on the Yin/Yang concept of meeting hard with soft, using leverage rather than muscle tension to neutralize attacks. The easily recognizable slow, gentle, flowing movements of Tai Chi have been seen in large crowds across China and around the world. It is often seen as a kind of moving meditation. It follows many of the principles of Traditional Chinese Medicine and has many reported health benefits, especially for the elderly. Researchers have found the long-term Tai Chi practice has favorable effects in balance, flexibility, cardiovascular fitness with reports of reduced pain, stress and anxiety in healthy subjects. It has also been shown to decrease falls in the elderly.

There are many different styles today but they're based on the system originally taught by the Chen family to the Yang family beginning in 1820. Training involves learning the solo routines called "forms". There is also advanced training known as "pushing hands" for two people and also weapons training. There are several major styles of Tai Chi, each named after the Chinese family where it originated. These are: Chen Style; Yang Style; Wu Style; Hao Style; Sun Style and Zhaobao Style. In 1956 the Chinese Sports Committee shortened the Yang Family form to 24 postures, often called the Short Form of Tai Chi. The longer traditional solo forms can have 88 to 108 postures. In 1976 a combination form called the Combined 48 Forms was created. Today there are dozens of new styles and hybrids which have grown out of the main styles.

In 1970 Taoist Tai Chi was introduced to the West by Master Moy Lin-Shin. This form is different because it is designed to promote and restore health. The Taoist Style uses greater stretching and turning in all of the movements to increase the benefits of Tai Chi.

There is no universal certification process for Tai Chi so almost anyone can call themselves a teacher. As with all exercise programs it is wise to first check with your physician and also carefully research the training and experience of the Tai Chi instructor.

In the 2007 federal government survey of CAM Tai Chi was researched as a separate type of mind-body therapy. There were 2,267 responses that Tai Chi had been used in the previous year for a 1.0% rate.

`https://nccih.nih.gov/health/taichi, http://www.wustyle.com/site/`

USER COMMENTS:

♦ The first thought I had was 'How hard can it be to learn 24 moves?' As it turns out, it can take a lifetime. An impatient American can learn the fundamentals of the moves in a few weeks or months but the subtleties, the wonderful delicate touches, can take years.

♦ I signed up for the class because I loved the grace of the movements and needed some serious stress reduction in my life. This moving meditation as it's called seemed ideal. It looks easy but the effects are amazing. There is a feeling of peace and freedom after doing Tai Chi that is difficult to explain. It looks easy but it can feel like a workout when you're done, but it also relaxes the body and the mind in a unique way. For those of us with limited muscle memory it means practicing regularly or it's like starting all over again!

TIBETAN MEDICINE

Today's **Tibetan Medicine** comes from an ancient form of healing called ***Gso-wa Rig-pa*** or "The Knowledge of Healing" which is estimated to go back nearly 4,000 years. The foundation of this medical system is that balance among the physical, psychological and spiritual facets of human existence produce health.

In addition to their own medical wisdom about the 4th century Tibetans began adding features of other systems as well including Ayurveda from India. In the 7th and 8th centuries they added elements from China, Persia and Greece to their base of knowledge. By the 11th century they synthesized these principals of physical and psychological healing with a distinctly Buddhist spiritual perspective into a unique system of medicine. In 1961 the 14th Dalai Lama built the Tibetan Medical and Astro-Institute at Dharamsala, India to preserve their medical knowledge and the Tibetan culture.

We cannot achieve good health just by being physically healthy; we also have to have a healthy mind. The mind and the five elements (fire, earth, etc.) manifest themselves in the form of body, energy and mind. These are reflected in the three basic systems of the body which are translated into English as Wind, Bile and Phlegm. These three systems are supposed to create and maintain all of the body's functions. For example, the Wind system deals with blood circulation and the movement of nerve impulses.

In Tibetan Medicine illness is the result of ignorance. Because we don't understand the nature of reality we act in ways that cause problems. Tibetan doctors begin by examining patients in a variety of ways including urinalysis, the taking of pulses along with observing the tongue, eyes and even the sensitivity of certain pressure points. Physicians then start treatment by recommending behavioral and lifestyle changes. If additional therapy is needed they progress to dietary treatments. If the patient requires even more help they use herbal medicines and then physical therapies like acupuncture. Prescription drugs and surgery are used only as a last resort.

Please carefully investigate the education and training of any health practitioner, especially one based on a foreign culture, along with required licensing and certifications to practice in your area.

`www.tibetanmedicine.com/index.html,`

`www.takingcharge.csh.umn.edu/explore-healing-practices/tibetan-medicine`

TRAGER® APPROACH

The **Trager® Approach** uses gentle, natural movements to produce deep relaxation and increased physical mobility. Underlying physical and mental patterns which may have developed from accidents, illness or other trauma are also released with this process. It uses movement education for mind-body integration to produce long-lasting effects. Some people use this technique for personal growth. The approach had also been known as Trager Work or Trager Psychophysical Integration and is more approach than specific treatment process.

Dr. Milton Trager discovered the principles of his technique as a teenaged boxer when he intuitively accessed a style of bodywork while giving a rubdown to his trainer. Surprised by the experience he applied it to his father and after just two sessions managed to clear up his father's chronic sciatica. Dr. Trager spent the next 50 years refining and expanding his discovery to learn more about the effects of these gentle movements on the nervous system and the unconscious mind.

There are two different aspects of The Trager® Approach which complement each other. The first is a passive technique called tablework where the client is lying on a comfortable table. Before each session the trained practitioner enters into a meditative state called "hook up" to better communicate with the client's body. Then the practitioner supports and moves the client in normal ways but with a touch that provides the sensation of effortless motion. Sessions normally last 60 to 90 minutes and the client is dressed comfortably but with a minimum of clothing.

Mentastics® (short for mental and gymnastics) is the active portion of The Trager Approach®, taught in both private and group sessions. The instructions for these simple movements teach clients how to take care of themselves and relieve stress on their own during daily activities. These self-induced movements reinforce the quality of effortless movement developed during the tablework.

Beginning in 1980 the Trager Institute and today the United States Trager Association's certification program requires at least 409 hours of training normally taking at least six months to complete. The 2007 survey reported just 37 respondents on this therapy.

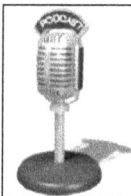

I spoke with Roger Tolle, spokesman for the United States Trager Association and an instructor and practitioner for more than 20 years about this approach to helping others. Roger studied with the creator of the process, Dr. Milton Trager, and today he spreads the word about this unique process in both English and German.

`www.trager.com or http://www.tragerus.org/`

USER COMMENTS:

♦ Trager® has been the most memorable and life-altering experience I have had in healthcare. From the ages of 19 through 30, I was consistently in physical pain, unable to be helped by various forms of treatment including cortisone treatments, muscle relaxers, chiropractic, massage, meditation and hypnosis. I was finally diagnosed with muscular rheumatism, told I would have to learn to relax and accept a slower lifestyle. I remember as if it was today, my third Trager Session... I stood up off the table, free of pain, with a sense of a new body. Like all people, I do experience occasional pain, but for the last 25 years, and today at 55, I live a very active lifestyle without daily pain. Thanks to that Trager session and the Trager exercises, Mentastics®, I can bring back the feelings of freedom, relax and know I am not trapped by pain. It is that freedom that led me to become a Trager Practitioner, helping my clients... and delighted to hear them say 'Trager is amazing, I don't have that pain anymore.'

♦ My chronic shoulder pain was treated with cortisone injections and with many physical therapy visits, but Trager® eliminated the pain and gave me more range of motion.

♦ I don't know that I've ever felt as relaxed as I was on your table. My memory of it is certainly like floating on a cloud. The residual effects have left me calmer and clearer. I had been having trouble relaxing, especially when it was time to do so. Since my session with you, I'm able to recall the feelings and sink in, allowing myself to rest onto that cloud. The Mentastics®, too, continue to help me practice relaxing my muscles. I can certainly see how successive sessions would build and reinforce the sensory memory.

TTOUCH-For-You

TTouch-For-You is the human therapeutic adaptation of the **Tellington Touch** animal therapy developed by Linda Tellington-Jones in 1983. She developed the therapy after training with Dr. Moshe Feldenkrais (see **Feldenkrais® Method**). While owners were learning the therapy for their animals they'd experiment on each other and the benefits of the therapy for people quickly became clear.

This is a system of circular motions, lifts and slides that works to activate the body's healing potential at the cellular level. There are twenty different types of TTouches including Ear TTouches, Hair Slides, Heart Tug and Octopus, often using small circular motions. One example is The Hair Pulling Slide technique that applies gentle pressure, moving in the direction away from the scalp to the ends of small sections of hair. The movement creates pressure at and beneath the scalp which is quite pleasurable and relaxing. The process can lower your pulse rate and blood pressure, slow respiration and neutralize stress chemicals in the body associated with the "fight or flight" response.

Linda Tellington-Jones co-authored *Massage And Physical Therapy For The Athletic Horse* based on the teachings of her grandfather, William Caywood. Her latest books are *The Tellington TTouch: Caring for Animals With Heart And Hands* and *TTouch for Healthcare*.

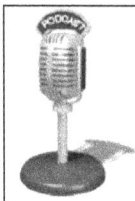

Linda Tellington-Jones originally created TTouch for horses but quickly discovered its benefits for people. She is an internationally recognized authority on animal behavior, training and healing. Linda is also Founder and President of TTouch Training. Our conversation on the health benefits of TTouch shows how much we have in common with our animal friends.

www.tteam-ttouch.com

USER COMMENTS:

♦ I recently flew to Indiana for a week to be with my parents. My father is 88 years old and has Alzheimer's. He was talking gibberish. Not one word was intelligible, just a string of syllables. I put both hands on his bald head and began Lying Leopard TTouches, very slowly. He was suddenly silent. For about 2 or 3 minutes, I continued all over his head. Then I sat down. He began talking in well-articulated words and sentences! My mom was amazed!

♦ A client of mine has found a way to reduce the most wearing symptoms of his Multiple Sclerosis to a minimum with Tellington-TTouch For You®. It has improved his quality of life significantly. He is still incurably ill but his worst symptoms have decreased so much that he has found a new interest in everything. He is also cheerful again—according to his wife he is almost the same person he was before the disease spread in his body. He himself confirms 'Today I enjoy life again!'

♦ I fell 9-½ feet off a stair landing and landed on a concrete sidewalk on my left hip. I endured months of pain, limited mobility, side effects of pain pills and a generally deteriorating quality of life. I felt like a piece of beef with little connectedness to my doctors or the physical therapist. When I first experienced a session of Tellington TTouch I was pretty desperate, experiencing a significant amount of chronic pain, and in an emotionally dark and hopeless place.

♦ Our TTouch session was not like any other type of body work I have received. I appreciated how much you checked in with how I felt as you worked with me. It helped me to understand that TTouch is really something you do WITH the person, not just TO them. While I felt relaxed after our session, I also felt energized and decided to go out for a walk. I was surprised that I felt good enough to climb up and down a very long flight of stairs at my local park and still my knee felt great. My knee hasn't felt that good since I injured it. Thank you for the time you spent with me. I'd like to schedule another session as much for the feeling of calm well being I had as for the benefit of my knee.

TUINA (also TUI-NA)

Tuina or **Tui Na** is referred to as Chinese Medical Massage and is a basic part of Traditional Chinese Medicine. The words Tui Na translate into "push-grasp" or "poke-pinch" in Chinese. It's a form of deep-tissue massage that's used to relieve chronic pain and a range of common ailments. The therapy is based on Taoist and martial arts principles to bring the energy of the body into balance for better health.

Practitioners use a variety of techniques to get the energy or chi moving in the meridians and muscles. They may brush, knead, roll, press or rub the areas between each of the joints known as the eight gates in TCM to remove blockages and open the flow of energy using palms, fingertips, knuckles or tools. Afterwards they may use traction and range of motion techniques along with the stimulation of acupressure points as part of the process. Sessions can last from ten minutes to more than an hour. It's beneficial for both acute and chronic musculoskeletal conditions but has a reputation for being a powerful, but quite painful, therapy. There is also self-Tuina techniques and now Sports Tuina for athletes.

As with many ancient Chinese therapies there were a variety of forms and traditions but the late Dr. Da-fang Yu is often credited with the integration of the forms into a systemized standard called Modern Orthodox Tui-Na today.

As with many of these therapies with a variety of forms it's best to ask about the education and training of your practitioner prior to treatment.

`www.tui-na.com`

WATSU® or Water Shiatsu

Watsu® therapy is one of the early forms of aquatic bodywork. It combines elements of shiatsu, muscle stretching, massage and dance with graceful, fluid movements in a warm water environment. Working in water requires the client be supported at all times which creates a connection between therapist and client that is much deeper than work done on a table. The therapeutic benefits of warm water include greater freedom of movement and deep relaxation.

The technique was developed in 1980 by Harold Dull, a Northern California massage therapist. After returning from Japan he began floating his **Zen Shiatsu** students in the warm water of Harbin Hot Springs. The idea of stretching to open the flow of energy channels is even older than acupuncture. Stretching also strengthens muscles and increases flexibility. The support provided by working in warm water relieves compression in joints like vertebrae and decreases muscle tension allowing movement that is not possible out of the water.

In addition to traditional Watsu® there are three major styles: **Waterdance; Healing Dance** and the **Jahara Technique.** The Waterdance technique is done completely beneath the surface. The Healing Dance style is a mix between regular Watsu and Waterdance. The Jahara Technique is called the gentlest form because of its constant support and gentle bodywork. One of the common features are moments of stillness alternated with rhythmical, flowing movements, often using the Water Breath Dance which is the rising and falling back caused by each breath. Originally Watsu® involved a therapist supporting the client but with the use of floatation devices today there is a greater range of movement possible. Sessions are usually 50-60 minutes but can vary depending on your therapist and health condition.

Watsu® is practiced in more than 40 countries and is accepted as a key methodology in rehabilitation by aquatic therapists. The Worldwide Aquatic Bodywork Association (WABA) supervises Watsu® standards along with maintaining a registry of authorized practitioners. Since this is considered a type of massage, please check with your state regarding regulations and certifications in your area.

www.waba.edu

USER COMMENTS:

♦ You've never really been relaxed until you've had a Watsu session! After trying massage and even Rolfing, Watsu was recommended to help me relax so the muscles could heal better. Floating in warm water (in my case it happened to be saltwater for added buoyancy) while wearing floatation devices on my legs, arms and around my waist and head produced a totally weightless sensation. It took a few minutes for me to actually relax and not worry about drowning but the calming words of the therapist helped guide me through the process.

♦ The movements are slow and gentle and sometimes you can barely tell you're moving at all. Stretches start small and grow as your muscles adapt. There are motions possible floating in water that just can't be done on a massage table, and they're wonderful.

♦ The slow breathing and constant support of the therapist brought back memories of being cradled in my mother's arms as a baby. The relaxation that you feel after a Watsu session is incredible, like a massage and hot tub rolled together.

♦ The mother of an 11-year-old boy with ankylosing spondylitis (arthritis of the spine) witnessed that peace (from Watsu) in her pain-ridden child. The disease, which causes severe pain in the joints, was prevalent in the boy's back and hips. He was also diagnosed with attention deficit hyperactivity disorder (ADHD). Getting treatments three to four times a week with Watsu seemed to reduce his negative behaviors, especially through the eyes of his mother, the nurses and staff.

TIP

The River of Renewal/flows across the land/from the rapids of advice/to the ocean's warm sands./ Plot your course with great care/and soon you will find/a destination of better health/for body and mind./ Friends and family may drown you with advice/but avoid the rocks, don't pay the price. / *Instead steer with care/keep an eye on the shore/and soon you will find/great health is your score.*

YOGA

In the U.S. **yoga** is considered mainly a form of exercise concentrating on postures (asanas) and breathing. The rest of the world recognizes yoga as a means for both physical health and spiritual mastery. Yoga connects the movement of the body with the rhythm of the breath and the mind. According to the 2002 survey of CAM practices by the federal government 7.5% of Americans have ever used yoga and 5.1% used it in the previous 12 months. The 2007 survey showed the prior year's use increasing to 6.1%. Yoga Journal magazine's 2005 survey estimates there are 16.5 million yoga practitioners in the U.S. today.

Yoga is a collection of ancient spiritual practices originating in India for integrating mind, body and spirit to achieve oneness with the universe. While it is one of the schools of Hindu philosophy it is a spiritual practice, not a religion, and it does not require any specific beliefs for participation. Yoga is also central to Buddhism, Tibetan Buddhism, Jainism and has influenced many other religions.

A male who practices yoga is a yogi, and a female practitioner is a yogini. While there is a lot of crossover between yoga schools and variations within each style there are many common features. Hatha yoga is the most popular style in the U.S. today. It was introduced in the 15ᵗʰ century as an outgrowth of an older style known as Raja yoga. It's used to prepare the body for higher meditation. Because it develops health and flexibility, students in the U.S. are usually not interested in the complete Hatha yoga process which deals with spiritual development.

Hatha represents opposing energies such as hot and cold, male and female, in a similar fashion to the Chinese concept of yin and yang. It works to balance the mind and body by physical exercises called asanas using controlled breathing, and the calming of the mind through relaxation and meditation. These postures develop balance, strength and reduce stress.

It is important to find both a yoga style and yoga teacher that you're comfortable with for the best results. The traditional instructions for Hatha yoga include having a glass of fresh water before the session. The asanas should be done on an empty stomach to prevent discomfort, and are best done in the early morning. Asanas should not involve force or pressure and movements should be slow and gentle. Breathing should always be done through the nose and in a controlled manner. Yoga should be done in a peaceful, clean, well-lit room that is well ventilated.

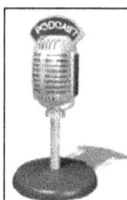

> Yoga has become one of the most popular therapies in America with nearly 16 million adults participating in this ancient form of exercise. I spoke with Elizabeth Winter, Assistant Editor of *Yoga Journal* magazine and yoga practitioner for 6 years, about the health benefits and the features of yoga.

https://en.wikipedia.org/wiki/Yoga
www.yogajournal.com

Ananda Yoga is a way to release unwanted tensions and to grow spiritually. This system uses silent affirmations while holding a posture, a technique intended to deepen and enhance the subtle benefits of each asana. This is a technique for aligning the body, its energy, and the mind with a series of gentle postures created to move energy upward to the brain.

www.expandinglight.org/anandayoga/

Anusara Yoga® is said to mean, "stepping into the current of divine will." This new system developed by John Friend **blends** the human spirit with the science of biomechanics. It is different from other yoga systems by three features: Attitude; Alignment and Action.

www.anusara.com

Ashtanga Yoga is a system of six, fast-paced series of sequential postures of increasing difficulty which is why sweating comes easily.

www.ashtanga.com

Bikram Yoga is also called hot yoga because room temperatures can be near 100° Fahrenheit. This environment helps move toxins out of the body by sweating. There is a series of 26 traditional Hatha postures directed at each body system.

www.bikramyoga.com

Hatha Yoga is often a blending of different styles of yoga under what has become almost a generic banner. This being the case, it's probably a good idea to check into the class to see if it's more in the meditative or active style before signing up. It might not hurt to check into the teacher's training and experience too.

www.yogajournal.com/category/yoga-101/types-of-yoga/hatha/

Integral Yoga is the form of yoga Sri Swami Satchidananda developed in 1966 to help people integrate the teachings of yoga into their everyday life. This is to promote greater peace and tolerance in the individual.

Integrative Yoga Therapy was introduced in 1993 in San Francisco by Joseph Le Page, M.A. This is a yoga teacher-training program designed specifically for medical environments such as hospitals and rehabilitation centers.

www.iytyogatherapy.com

Iyengar Yoga puts an intense focus on the subtleties of each position by requiring students to hold each position longer. Students can pay close attention to the precise muscular and skeletal alignment this system demands with this longer attention. The system also uses props such as belts and chairs to deal with special needs such as injuries.

www.bksiyengar.com

Jivamukti Yoga is a highly meditative form of yoga that is also physically challenging. Sessions may include chanting, meditation, readings, music, and affirmations along with the postures.

www.jivamuktiyoga.com

Kali Ray Tri Yoga® was created in 1980 as a new flowing method of yoga. Tri Yoga fundamentals include relaxation-in-action, wave-like spinal movements and economy of motion. With the systematic approach students can remain with Basics or progress to subsequent levels. Music accompanies the classes ending with meditation.

www.triyoga.com

Kundalini Yoga was a secret process that came from the Tantra yoga path until Yogi Brahan introduced it to the West in 1969. It is supposed to help seekers of enlightenment from all religious paths tap into their greater potential. This system uses postures and dynamic breathing techniques along with chanting and meditating on mantras. Students focus on awakening the energy at the base of the spine and drawing it upward through each of the traditional seven chakras.

https://www.3ho.org/kundalini-yoga

Phoenix Rising Yoga Therapy is a synthesis of traditional yoga and contemporary body-mind psychology which can produce a release of physical tensions and emotional blocks.

www.pryt.com

Power Yoga was a term Beryl Bender Birch created to describe Ashtanga yoga to Americans. It's a workout of a series of poses designed not to create heat and energy flow but to serve as a traditional methodology for spiritual transformation. Because of the athletic and powerful nature of the physical portion of the system it's popular in health clubs and gyms.

www.power-yoga.com

Sahaja Yoga is a method of meditation created in 1970 to bring a new level of awareness. The process is supposed to help you experience the power of the divine as your awareness expands. As a result students become more integrated and balanced, capable of effortless spiritual growth.
www.sahajayoga.org/

Sivananda Yoga is a path to learn about who you really are. It is supposed to help you appreciate each level of experience.
www.sivananda.org

Svaroopa® Yoga teaches different ways of doing familiar poses. It focuses on opening the spine by beginning at the tailbone and progressing through each area. This is a consciousness-oriented yoga that also promotes healing which many consider a very approachable style.
www.svaroopa.org/

Tibetan Yoga is composed of five flowing movements. It is an active workout that features constant motion. Students may begin with 10 or 12 repetitions and work their way up to the 21 repetitions of the full routine.
www.tibetanyoga.com/

Viniyoga is a practice designed to work on all levels. The poses are synchronized with the breath. It is a process for developing a style to meet each person's needs as they grow.
www.viniyoga.com

White Lotus Yoga is a flowing style that varies from gentle to vigorous depending on ability and comfort level. Classes involve alignment, breath, and the theories of yoga.
www.WhiteLotus.org

ZEN BODYTHERAPY® or Zentherapy®

Zentherapy® is the belief that life is the flow of energy called Ki or Chi. As we live and grow, this life-force energy shapes our emotions and bodies. Zentherapy® releases the changes caused by physical, psychological and spiritual traumas so the natural form of the body can return. By releasing the traumas held in the body, the mind and spirit also change.

William S. ("Dub") Leigh developed the process as a result of his studies with three masters. He learned about the structure of the body from Ida Rolf and about function from Moshe Feldenkrais. In Hawaii he trained under Zen Master and martial artist Tanouye Tenshin Rotaishi, a healer adept at the use of Ki. By combining the deep-tissue work of Rolfing®, the body re-education of the Feldenkrais Method® along with the energy training of Tanouye Rotaishi, he created a unique new process.

The International Zentherapy® Institute, Inc. is headquartered in Hawaii and is the only source for training and certification in this modality. As a form of bodywork, practitioners must have massage licensing in most states.
www.zentherapy.org

BODY DEVICES

COLD LASER THERAPY or Low Level Laser Therapy (LLLT) or Cold Laser Acupuncture

The use of light for healing goes back thousands of years but the process is growing in popularity with the latest technology. Light or photon energy with limited power, a few J/cm2 with laser power of 50 mW or less, penetrates up to two inches below the surface of the skin with no tissue damage. There is no heat or pain from this type of device and it is being used to treat a variety of health problems.

The FDA first approved the use of **cold laser therapy** to treat neck and shoulder pain, following with approval for carpal tunnel syndrome in 2002, however most insurance companies deny coverage considering the technology experimental. These devices are also being used to treat a variety of inflamed conditions of soft tissues and joints such as sports injuries, arthritis, back pain and other injuries to the musculoskeletal system. Cold lasers are even being used as "pointless" acupuncture, using light energy to stimulate the acupuncture points without pain and to stimulate lymph drainage. One of the most popular cold laser acupuncture treatments is to help stop smoking. Cold lasers are even being used to stimulate hair follicles to prevent hair loss and promote hair growth.

One type of device is **Anodyne® Therapy** which comes from the word anodyne, meaning a medical treatment that soothes or relieves pain. This device uses monochoromatic near-infrared photo energy (MIRE) with pads that emit the light being applied to the surface of the skin. The technique usually focuses on the feet, often those with diabetes or PAD. It was approved by the FDA and first used in 1994.

http://en.wikipedia.org/wiki/Low_level_laser_therapy
www.erchonia.com

USER COMMENTS:

- This (cold laser) unit has been an invaluable tool in helping us treat our veteran patients who suffer from chronic pain and chronic non-healing ulcers. Before we had this unit, we were treating chronic pain patients with regular processes including moist heat, TENS and microcurrent. We have had moderate success in reducing patients' pain with these processes. With the unit we have had significant reduction in pain levels when treating our chronic pain patients. We have had some patients' pain levels decrease to almost zero (on a 10-point scale) after one or two treatments. This includes patients with such painful conditions as diabetic neuropathy and dry gangrene.

- I have been in practice for over 35 years working in the field of head, neck and facial pain. There is no question in my mind that this laser is the one and only modality that a physical therapist needs in his tool box.

- Too often we think that what we can't see won't hurt us. Wrong! While going through physical therapy for a back injury, the therapist decided to use a cold laser treatment to promote healing. There was a chart on the wall of what points they're supposed to use, but apparently she had decided that since it was "painless" that it would be okay to just run it all up and down the back muscles to stimulate healing.

It also stimulated every acupuncture point in my back! The result was that I didn't sleep for nearly two days because my system was over-stimulated and pumped full of adrenaline. Everyone really needs to learn about the specific machine being used, the training the operator has had, their results (and problems) and be very, very careful.

HYPERBARIC OXYGEN THERAPY (HBOT)

Hyperbaric Oxygen Therapy or HBOT refers to treating the body with 100% oxygen at higher than normal pressure. The term comes from "hyper" meaning increased and "baric" which relates to pressure. Normally we breathe 20% oxygen at one atmospheric absolute, which is abbreviated as ATA. With HBOT pure oxygen is given at up to two times normal pressure either in an individual or group chamber. This combination of increased oxygen and pressure results in pushing oxygen for healing into the blood, fluids and body tissues at up to twenty times normal levels.

Originally the technique was developed to help skin divers recover from surfacing too quickly, a condition known as "the bends", but the benefits of HBOT have been demonstrated on a wide variety of health problems. Pressurized oxygen has been especially beneficial for neurological problems such as cerebral palsy, brain injury, Multiple Sclerosis and stroke. HBOT has also been used successfully to treat peripheral vascular disease, burns, diabetic ulcers, carbon monoxide poisoning and macular degeneration. HBOT can help restore function and increase healing whenever blood flow and oxygen delivery has been compromised. Treatments usually last between an hour to an hour-and-a-half but 50 to 100 treatments may be required for full effect.

While accepted by many in the mainstream medical community the therapy is not widely used, possibly due lack of physician familiarity. It's estimated that less than 20% of the medical schools in the country have their own hyperbaric oxygen facility and perhaps only 15% or 20% more may have access to one. Simply put, if doctors aren't trained or don't know about a therapy then they're reluctant to prescribe it. This chicken-and-egg situation is a common problem with complementary and alternative therapies.

The cost for a single HBOT treatment session may vary from $150 to nearly $1,000 per hour. Medicare did approve HBOT for the treatment of diabetic foot wounds in 2003 but most insurance companies deny coverage because the FDA has not issued a formal approval due to a lack of research. It costs millions of dollars to conduct the necessary research for FDA approval but since oxygen can't be patented the profit potential is limited. Without FDA approval and subsequent insurance reimbursement there is limited interest in developing new HBOT facilities. This is a common problem with CAM therapies.

www.hyperbaricmedicalassociation.org

LIGHT THERAPY or Phototherapy

Light Therapy or **phototherapy** is normally associated with treatment of a particular type of depression known as **seasonal affective disorder** or SAD, also called winter depression. Exposure to bright lights reduces the brain's production of melatonin which controls the body's internal clock, reducing the effects of SAD. Recommendations are for at least two hours of sunlight each day for good physical and emotional health.

Treatment is done with special fixtures which produce bright light, normally up to twenty times light levels in an office or home. Originally full-spectrum bulbs were used because they most closely resembled natural light but some research suggests that brightness is more important than color spectrum. Treatment products produce light ranging from 2,500 to 10,000 lux and exposure times will vary from up to two hours with lower power units to approximately 30 minutes with high-powered devices. Exposure is usually recommended first thing in the morning to help reset

"Isn't it amazing how just a little improvement can add so much hope?"

- Karen

the body's clock to a spring day. While light therapy may be used in the evening for severe cases, it can also interfere with normal sleep patterns. Clocks which mimic normal sunrise, called Dawn Clocks, are also used to treat SAD.

Light Therapy is also used to treat jet lag since it can be useful in resetting the body's clock. Other types of light therapy are used to treat acne, psoriasis and eczema. Full-spectrum lighting is used to treat neonatal jaundice (bilirubin).

Another type of light therapy is called Solar Therapy or Heliotherapy and decades ago it was used to treat tuberculosis. The winner of the second Nobel Prize for Medicine in 1903 was awarded to Dr. Niels Finsen for his work with the therapy and creation of the Finsen Lamp. Sunlight was also used as an antibiotic and therapy during World War I.

There are other types of Light Therapy that are considered a type of vibrational medicine for use on acupuncture points or meridians, chakras or other areas (see **Gem Therapy**). In these situations specific colors of light are used to stimulate energy centers to improve energy flow. Since light is a type of energy it's believed that different colors have healing effects on the body's energy system.

Standard Light Therapy has been used to treat SAD since the 1980s but is not approved by the FDA due to a shortage of effective research. If your doctor prescribes Light Therapy your insurance may cover the cost but it is recommended you check with your carrier first. Light boxes may be purchased over-the-counter but it is recommended you discuss treatment with your doctor since there are risks involved including eye damage.

www.mayoclinic.com/health/seasonal-affective-disorder/DS00195

PERCUTANEOUS ELECTRICAL NERVE STIMULATION (PENS) also Percutaneous Neuromodulation Therapy (PNT)

A single event of back pain can cause the nerve cells to become hypersensitive, a condition which can continue long after the original injury has healed. In addition to TENS therapy (*see listing this section*) there are additional pain relief therapies like **Percuntaneous Electrical Nerve Stimulation** (PENS) and **Percutaneous Neuromodulation Therapy** (PNT). Both are low-risk therapies relying on inserting fine needles through the skin, similar to electrical acupuncture, but placement is not determined by energy meridians as it is with Traditional Chinese Medicine.

For those patients who cannot find back pain relief with TENS therapy, these therapies offer additional hope for a non-surgical pain solution. TENS effectiveness can be reduced or eliminated by obesity, scar tissue and other barriers to electrical stimulation. Both PENS and PNT are based on inserting fine-gauge electrodes (about 250 microns in diameter) to a depth of 1 to 4 cm with electrical stimulation of 15 to 30 Hz. PENS placement is located around the painful area so placement is guided by the location of the pain. By comparison PNT therapy places up to 10 electrodes at specific locations in the back. Treatment protocols are for 30-minute sessions up to three times per week for up to ten sessions.

Both types of treatment devices have been approved by the Food and Drug Administration (FDA) for patients suffering from chronic low back or neck pain. In addition there are clinical trials underway at the National Center for Complementary and Alternative Medicine (NCCAM) and the National Institute of Aging (NIA) which are still listed as "active - not recruiting" at this time.

http://www.spine-health.com/treatment/pain-management/percutaneous-neuromodulation-therapy-pnt

PULSED-ELECTROMAGNETIC FIELD THERAPY (PEMF)

Pulsed Electromagnetic Field Therapy (PEMF) is based on the principle that the human body is electrical as well as chemical and that particular frequencies can have healing effects on wounds and disease. The original technology which created negative polarity with electromagnetic waves was developed in the 1930s. One of the earliest research studies was conducted at the Scripps Ranch in 1934 by Milbank Johnson, M.D., Arthur I. Kendall, Ph.D., Professor of Bacteriology at Northwestern University Medical School, E.C. Rosenow Sr., Director of Research at the Mayo

Clinic in Rochester, and Royal R. Rife. Their conclusions were that Rife's electromagnetic generator (*also see* **Rife Technology**) either interrupted the reproductive ability of viruses, bacteria and parasites or simply destroyed the pathogens. Tumors were also reported to shrink when exposed to negative polarity.

One machine was developed by Abraham Ginsburg, M.D. and physicist Arthur Milinowski in 1932 but had difficulty becoming accepted until the technology was used successfully to help burns and other wounds heal faster following the Israeli-Arab war in 1967. However in 1972 the FDA stepped in and banned all of the devices, a move that was reversed by a 1987 court order that found the FDA had been "arbitrary and capricious". The technology is currently FDA approved for use for post-operative swelling and pain in soft tissue.

Current models focus electromagnetic energy to a specific body area through a cylindrical treatment head mounted on a moveable arm. The energy easily penetrates clothing, casts, or bandages and has no known side effects.

Because these devices pulse their electromagnetic output, they emit energy for only a fraction of time, allowing any heat associated with the transferred energy to dissipate. Although considered experimental by most insurance companies there are research studies from around the world demonstrating the effectiveness of the principle.

`www.scribd.com/doc/13683959/History-of-Pulsed-Electro-Magnetic-Field-Therapy`

RIFE TECHNOLOGY or Resonant Frequency Therapy

Rife Technology, Rife/Bare Device or **Resonant Frequency Therapy** is a device to produce an electromagnetic wave to put healing energy into the body. The technology is based on the concept that every living entity, including a cancer virus, resonates a unique bio-energy frequency. This device produces specific healing frequencies for each type of illness or disease.

The original device was created by Dr. Royal Raymond Rife in the 1930s to emit energy that would kill a cancer virus inside patients. He was an accomplished scientist and invented the most powerful microscope of its day. There are many stories, almost legends, about his successful medical tests with the Rife Device before it was attacked by the American Medical Association and the California State Medical Society. By 1939 the device had fallen into disfavor and much of the information about the technology was lost for decades.

Today a new version of Resonant Frequency Therapy is available with the Rife/Bare Device which produces four times the amount of electromagnetic energy per watt from improved electronics. Devices may be purchased over the Internet or assembled from do-it-yourself plans.

The list of frequencies for various diseases and illnesses has also improved over the years.

The technology is not FDA approved and no medical claims are made by any manufacturer to avoid problems with the FDA. Currently they claim the devices can only be sold in America for veterinary use, equipment testing and for personal investigation into the effects of frequencies. The FDA is researching the technology for food safety since it kills pathogens without harming tissue. Currently several universities are researching laser technologies that are incredibly close to Rife's "beam ray device" from decades earlier. You can learn more about Rife Technology by joining one of the Internet user groups like Yahoo's "Rife" group.

`www.rife.de, www.rife.org`

USER COMMENTS:

♦ I have had chronic euticaria on my forearms for the past five years. I have been prescribed medicines which are usually steroids and actizinone cream or phisoderm type products. This usually helps the symptoms of itching and pustules, temporarily at least. My arms are full of pockmark scars from the pustules and blisters that have come and gone over the past years.

I ran the device for approx 20 minutes. My arms did not itch for three more days and the pustules started to recede. After the third day I used a euticaria frequency from another database. All the pustules are gone and healed and I haven't experienced any more itching or pain.

I am so happy that something finally worked. Even the dermatologist could not figure out what was causing the condition. But after all methods of treatment failed, yours cured me. Thank you for making the technology available to those of us out here that really need and appreciate your efforts on our behalf.

♦ She was diagnosed with non-Hodgkin's lymphoma several years ago with obvious tumors in the lymph nodes. The tumors were slow growing, and the expected time of her death was 4-5 years in the future. Suggested treatment consisted of natural supplements to support the immune system and digestion with specific radionics charges for her conditions. Within a couple months, there was obvious improvement in all areas. At this writing, she reports that she is free of tumors. This has been confirmed by her MD.

TENS (Transcutaneous Electrical Nerve Stimulator)

TENS or **Transcutaneous Electrical Nerve Stimulator** is a pocket-sized electronic device that generates electrical signals to stimulate nerves through the skin for pain relief, frequently for the back. A typical unit is battery powered with controls for frequency and intensity, a pulse generator and transformer. The unit is connected by wires to electrodes which stick on the skin.

The TENS unit controls pain by sending electrical signals to the nerves blocking the pain signal to the brain. The positioning of the electrodes on the skin determines which muscles and nerves are stimulated. TENS may also work by stimulating the body's own endorphins in the brain which act to reduce pain.

Electrical stimulation for pain control actually goes back to ancient Greece. Early devices were developed back to the 16th century. Even Benjamin Franklin was a proponent of electricity for pain relief. Dr. C. Norman Shealy created a device called the dorsal column stimulator which contributed to the development of the TENS system. The modern, wearable TENS was patented in 1974 and was originally used for testing patient tolerance to electrical stimulation before a device was implanted in their spinal cord. Many of the patients got so much relief from the TENS unit that they never had the surgery.

The device is available from doctors, physical therapists, chiropractors and over the Internet. While it's possible to use a TENS unit for do-it-yourself experimentation it's beneficial to be trained in the best use of the device by an experienced professional.

`www.emedicine.com/pmr/topic206.htm`

USER COMMENTS:

♦ My chiropractor suggested I try a TENS during a particularly bad episode of lower back pain caused by bulging disks. This wasn't simply a backache but a down-on-your-hands-and-knees situation. I'd had back problems for years but this was one of the worst ones and I had a trade show coming up that was vital to my career. The idea of standing on concrete for several hours every day was almost enough to make me break out in a cold sweat.

You can't imagine the relief! It may sound painful but the little irritation of the low-powered TENS unit is nothing compared to the muscle and nerve pain of a bad back. I had to vary the intensity so my back didn't get too used to the sensation and begin to ignore it, but it worked wonderfully. By stimulating the muscles which had almost spasmed into concrete I was able to maintain enough flexibility to move around and function. What an incredible device! Wish I'd learned about it years ago.

> **TIP**
>
> An ocean of opportunities / is what you will find / as you progress down your path / in body and mind. / Health and vitality / joy and much more / are patiently waiting / it all can be yours.

BODY CATEGORY SUMMARY

The information in this book ran the gamut of human history from thousands of years ago (Ayurveda) to the newest inventions (Cold Laser and Pulsed Electromagnetic Field Therapy). You've seen therapies that deal with the entire body like Tai Chi and Rolfing to those that focus on specific problems like Lymph Drainage and Colonic Hydrotherapy.

By now your map is beginning to take shape. You've probably discovered many of the physical aspects of your own health issues and have made note of them on your map to help you find your way to better health. Like the landscape features we've covered each aspect on your personal map is unique. Each symptom that you have, every ache and pain, is part of your health scenery just like the mountains, rivers and forests are part of the world around you. Each one of these features offers unique challenges and opportunities.

Along the way you've also written down your experiences with different therapies along notes about what worked, and what didn't work so well. You've made note of your pitfalls and successes. You've noted the TIPS in this chapter to help you apply this map to your life. Your personal map is now beginning to fill in so it can help guide to you better health. Your map isn't blank any more! You really are making progress!

Perhaps you've even had great success with a particular body category therapy and discovered what it can do for your particular health problem. If the source of your health challenge was in the body hopefully you've found the right therapy for it. But remember, it may also only be a part of your problem. Some people are lucky to have easy single-source/single-therapy health issues. Most of us deal with more complicated situations. Instead of a single problem they may face a combination of issues that require a unique combination of therapies to resolve. Just like an old-fashioned combination lock, it can become much more challenging to unlock our natural ability to heal.

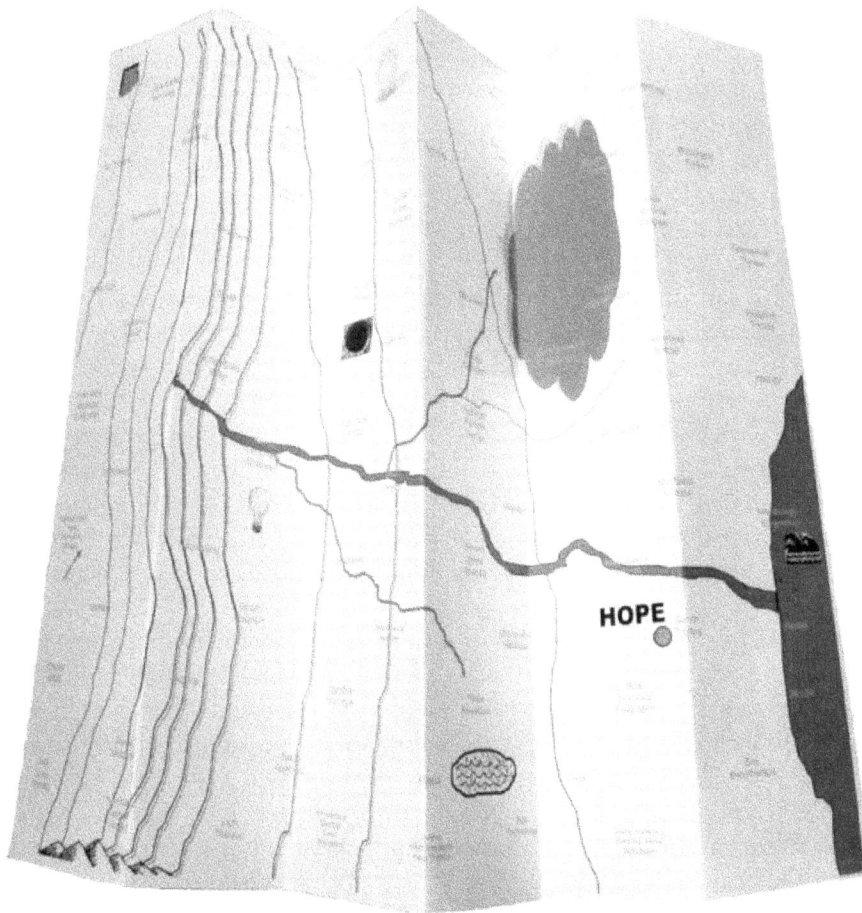

Chapter 3 – Insurance

Do you remember the old Jack Benny joke about him being robbed? Jack was walking down the street when a robber pulls him into an alley, points a gun at him and shouts "Your money or your life!" Jack rests his tilted head on his hand in his trademark posture, and after a few minutes the robber shouts again "I said your money or your life!" Jack shouts back "I'm thinking! I'm thinking!"

Thinking about insurance coverage and complementary and alternative therapies today feels a little bit like the Jack Benny joke. It can be about making tough choices. As patients and consumers we know how medical care has changed in this era of 8-minute appointments under managed care restrictions. Have you ever wondered why don't insurance companies don't seem to want cheaper, more effective treatments? Why doesn't America adopt a prevention-style health care system instead of the more expensive treatment approach?

Could part of the problem be that insurance companies want higher expenses so the states will approve higher premiums so they can make more money on the payment float and their investments? We know they'd rather pay $50,000 for a heart by-pass operation or $10,000 for a heart angioplasty operation than $150 for CAM methods to prevent problems even when they're medically proven and Medicare approved. To many people these look more like financial companies, not companies that care about the health of their customers. How else can you explain their reluctance to save money, lives and improve the quality of life for their customers?

Have you heard of the term "denial management" yet? It's one of the hot buzzwords in the healthcare debate going on today. Insurance companies make it a matter of policy to "deny-deny-

deny" claims submitted by doctors and hospitals for any minor infraction. Fact is, it's nearly impossible *not* to have a problem with every claim because doctors start out having to select the proper code out of up to 70,000 basic 5-digit codes. In addition each insurance company has their own constantly changing menu of codes and instructions like adding "-u5" to an established code to signify the latest update. It's a moving maze of delaying tactics that the insurance companies claim are designed to improve efficiencies and prevent fraudulent billing. The fact is that today this paperwork war is estimated to cost around $20 billion per year, about half from each side, in unnecessary administrative expenses according to a 2004 report by the Center for Information Technology Leadership.

Companies that are self-insured are beginning to realize the fundamental errors of our current system and are experiencing a paradigm shift in their attitudes. They're embracing wellness programs and health screenings because spending a little money up front saves big expenses later. In a 2006 *Wall Street Journal* article entitled "The Road To Wellness Is Starting At The Office" they reported on a recent survey by Hewitt Associates that found 42% of companies offered some type of health-risk assessment in 2005, up from 29% in 2001. Some companies are even setting up on-site clinics. In a follow-up article in 2009 titled "Get Well Or Pay Not To" the paper noted that 58% of U.S. companies now offer lifestyle improvement programs, up from 43% in 2007. The trend is to encourage employees to get healthy or charge them if they choose not to take advantage of available health programs.

While participation in corporate wellness programs is voluntary, many companies are beginning to shift to a surcharge for those workers who don't participate. Companies have a long-term incentive to encourage workers to participate in programs. Even though it usually takes two to five years for businesses to see the benefit, for every $1 they spend on programs they'll save $2 according to Hewitt Associates.

Be aware that most insurance companies and self-insured companies don't pay for complimentary or alternative therapies because they are classified as experimental or unproven even though they may have been around for thousands of years. This is one of the key factors restricting the growth of CAM therapies and it's a chicken-and-egg problem. Because most of these therapies cannot be patented like a drug there is limited profit potential, meaning there are no companies interested in investing millions of dollars for FDA testing. The National Center for Complementary and Alternative Medicine, a division of the National Institutes of Health, is involved with testing and research of these therapies but their budget is small compared to that of America's drug industry. Since NCCAM has only been in existence since 1999 they're still researching some of the oldest and most accepted therapies. Their research with the Mayo Clinic on the effectiveness of acupuncture for fibromyalgia was completed in 2005. At this rate it will be decades before many of the therapies listed here are evaluated properly.

There are some insurance companies beginning to pay for CAM treatments, usually for acupuncture, massage, chiropractic, biofeedback and naturopathy. Deductibles may also be higher than for regular medical care. A few insurance companies offer a special policy rider for CAM coverage so this may also be an option for you. Your insurance company may also have negotiated discounts with CAM therapy providers for a lower cost. It's best to discuss your coverage with your insurance carrier before beginning any new treatment. Even if your insurance company offers coverage they may require pre-authorization.

Some of the questions you may want to ask are:
- Do CAM treatments need to be pre-authorized or pre-approved?
- To obtain coverage do CAM treatments have to be authorized by prescription from a medical doctor?
- Do I need a referral for CAM from my primary care provider?
- Do I have to see only practitioners in your network to be covered?
- What coverage will I have if I use a practitioner out of network?
- Are there limits or restrictions on the number of visits or amount that you'll pay?

- ◆ What will my out-of-pocket expenses for CAM treatment be?
- ◆ Will my expenses for CAM treatments be included in my out-of-network deductible even if they're not covered?

Any time you deal with an insurance company it's wise to keep detailed records of every call and contact along with all bills, claims and letters. Also, it may take more than one CAM claim to get your insurance company to provide coverage. Keep trying! If it takes three, four, five claims or more ... keep pushing. It doesn't hurt to be persistent.

You may also want to contact your state's insurance department about coverage since there are many differences in state laws and policies. They may be able to help you find companies that offer better CAM coverage and what their ratings are for performance.

You may want to consider using a CAM practitioner who is part of a larger group. If nothing else if there are lab tests or other diagnostic tests needed you may be able to work with one of the regular physicians in the group to get coverage and they'll be more likely to prescribe CAM treatments for you.

On the other side of the issue there are also questions you should ask any potential CAM provider such as:

- • What does the first appointment cost?
- • What do follow-up appointments cost?
- • How many appointments are normally required?
- • Are there additional costs involved such as lab tests, equipment or supplements?
- • Do you take insurance?
- • What has your experience been dealing with insurance companies?
- • Do I file the insurance claim forms or will you take care of it?

If cost is an issue for you perhaps you can also ask if the practitioner offers a time payment option or a sliding fee scale.

If you are denied coverage for CAM treatment there are things that you can do. First of all, know your plan and exactly what it does, and does not, cover. You may also want to check and see if there is simply a clerical error in the coding. Compare the codes submitted on your practitioner's bill with the codes noted in the document from your insurance company. If you feel that your insurance company has made a mistake with your claim you can request a review because they all have a process for appealing denial of coverage. You can even ask your practitioner to support your efforts, for example, by preparing a letter to your insurance company. You can even file a complaint with your state's insurance agency regarding the problem.

There are new options to help with some CAM expenses like an FSA (Flexible Spending Arrangement) account. Some employers offer an FSA to help you put aside pretax dollars each pay period for health-related expenses. Some generous employers even make contributions to your account. You would submit receipts for expenses not covered by insurance for reimbursement. Be careful, in many cases the only expenses that can be covered are for treatments that are accepted by insurance companies according to the IRS.

For people who participate in a high-deductible health plan another option may be a Health Savings Account or HSA. This is another type of tax-exempt account you set up and maintain, although some employers may make contributions too. You're even allowed to invest your HSA monies to earn tax-deductible interest. For more information contact the IRS or check out www.irs.gov to learn more. Also note that beginning in the 2008 tax year the IRS allowed taxpayers to deduct medical expenses for a very limited number of CAM services and products. Please check with your tax preparation professional about this option. For more information check out IRS publication 969 - Health Savings Accounts and Other Tax-Favored Health Plans. There are also specific IRS publications available for particular options.

In some cases the federal government may help with some of the health expenses for CAM treatments. You'll need to check with each agency to learn about your benefits. Some assistance may be available from the Department of Veterans Affairs, Medicare or Medicaid (depending on your state's guidelines). The National Center for Complementary and Alternative Medicine does not provide financial assistance but it may be possible to participate in a clinical trial for a CAM therapy. To learn more you can visit

`https://nccih.nih.gov/research/clinicaltrials`

Chapter 4 – Conclusion

Don't you feel a new sense of hope after reading about all of these body-based complementary and alternative therapies? Doesn't it feel better to have a map to help you find the therapy you need for better health? Learning about all of these new and old options should open your eyes to the amazing possibilities that CAM has to offer you for better health and a better life. Just imagine how great you'll feel once you learn about all of the Mind and Energy/Spirit therapies! Millions of people around the world over thousands of years have proven that there are many different ways to *Unbreak Your Health*™ and treat the source of your problems, not just the symptoms. Robert Louis Stevenson said "Everyone who got where he is had to begin where he was" and that's the way it is with your search for better health. Now that you have a map and a sense of direction you can progress down your own path.

Almost everyone seems to know someone who's had a successful, even miraculous, experience with some type of complementary or alternative therapy. Once you begin talking with people about these opportunities you'll discover that you're not alone in your search for better health. You're part of a growing percentage of Americans determined to find better answers to their health questions. People may only have whispered about these techniques a few years ago but today the discussions are open and candid for one simple reason—they work, and they work without drugs. Effectiveness is the reason that a majority of Americans have used a complementary or alternative therapy today, even if they frequently come to it when the traditional medical community runs out of options.

There is a growing momentum to include complementary and alternative medicine as part of a shift to prevention in America's health care system. On February 26, 2009 the Senate Committee on Health, Education, Labor, and Pensions held a public hearing titled "Integrative Care: A Pathway to a Healthier Nation" which featured testimony from Dr. Mehmet Oz, Dr. Andrew Weil and Dr. Dean Ornish. The video of this hearing can be found at:

`http://www.help.senate.gov/hearings/-integrative-care-a-pathway-to-a-healthier-nation`

We're at the threshold of a new era of health and wellness, almost a Star Trek type of healing. The paradigm shift in medicine to using energy for healing instead of drugs has already started … very slowly, but the change is underway. We're slowly leaving the world of buggy whips and Newtonian science for the new age of quantum science and holistic health. There will always be those people and organizations that resist change but improvements for the better are inevitable.

The fact is the current U.S. sick-care system isn't working. U.S. health care spending grew 5.3 percent in 2014, reaching $3.0 trillion or $9,523 per person. As a share of the nation's Gross Domestic Product, health spending accounted for 17.5 percent, more than any other industrialized country. The U.S. only spends about $1.25 per person, less than 1% of the nation's healthcare budget, to prevent chronic diseases. Our healthcare results reflect our upside-down system and priorities.

The January 14, 2007 issue of *Parade* magazine reported that "We rank 30th in life expectancy for women and 28th for men. … (and) the U.S. position has steadily declined over the last 20 years." Since that time our ranking in the world has continued to decline, in 2009 we ranked 37th in the world.

We used to feel that America had the best medical system in the world. While that may not be the situation today the acceptance and legalization of complementary and alternative therapies may be one way to improve our health. It's time to explore all healthcare options today because we have too many people in this country who are sick and tired of being sick and tired.

Many of our doctors are the first to admit that mainstream medicine doesn't have all of the answers today and these are the ones most open to finding new ways to help their patients. There was a recent study of medical students at 126 medical schools across the country and 74% thought that a blend of Western medicine and CAM was better than either one alone so there is a fresh perspective entering the field. They accept that what they don't know far exceeds what they do know. They honestly try to know and understand their patients, even if it takes more than the time allotted by the managed care companies, because they sincerely want to be healers. These will be the leaders in the new world of medicine because they're open to all opportunities. They're interested only in the best possible results for each patient. These are the doctors leading the way in the movement to Integrative Medicine; they're part of the Consortium of Academic Health Centers for Integrative Medicine.

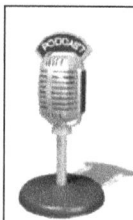

> It's no longer a black-or-white choice between CAM and mainstream medicine. The new trend is towards Integrative Medicine or utilizing the best of Eastern and Western medicine to meet the needs of each patient. I spoke with Eleanor D. Hynote M.D., a board certified internist, the Founder and Director of Phoenix Well Care in Napa, California and the President and CEO of the American College for Advancement in Medicine.

There are also doctors who will probably never change their mind, they'll always believe that drugs are the answer to everything, many of whom accept payments from drug companies. The *New England Journal of Medicine* reported in 2007 that their survey found 95% of doctors get gifts from drug sales representatives. The drug industry spends more than $20 billion per year on marketing nationwide. The *New York Times* reported that in Minnesota alone drug company payments to doctors increased from less than $2 million in 1997 to more than $12 million in 2004. Combined with the massive retail advertising done by the drug companies over the last few years to influence patients it's not surprising that our healthcare system is drug oriented.

Democrats and Republicans may have very different views of the world but both are valid from their point of view. Doctors are trained to see the human body as a bag of chemicals which is why their solutions usually involve drugs. Practitioners of complementary and alternative therapies view the human body as a complete being of mind, body and spirit/energy so they treat holistically. How you choose to "vote" on your healthcare will depend on your perspective and your particular problem but it's important to realize there are options. How can you make the most informed decision possible on your health care if you don't consider all of your options?

This book is about a new beginning, a better way to enjoy a healthy, vibrant life full of joy and vitality. It's about how you can *Unbreak Your Health*™ by finding the source of health problems instead of simply treating symptoms with drugs. YOU have the power to choose! YOU are the one responsible for your body and your life, but you have to become an aggressive patient and fight for yourself. If you want to treat a health problem this book offers many new options. If you want to become healthier to avoid illness this book offers many new possibilities in just one category, the body. This book, this map, is simply a tool, now it's *your* choice how best to use it to improve your life or to learn more about therapies in the Mind and Energy/Spirit categories.

I wish you more health and vitality, more joy and happiness.

—Alan E. Smith

Chapter 5 – Recommendations

"Protecting the public" has been the slogan used to prevent people from learning about healthcare opportunities outside the mainstream for too long. In 2014 preventable medical errors persisted as the No. 3 killer in the U.S. – third only to heart disease and cancer – claiming the lives of some 400,000 people each year. Can you imagine if 400,000 people died every year from one of the subjects in this book? Yet the medical community continues to stand on their pedestal and point a finger at all of the "unsafe" practices that they don't approve of claiming they're so dangerous that no one should be allowed to use them, regardless of how many centuries they've been practiced. They sound like any other type of business trying to protect their market share by any means possible.

The good news is that health care reform efforts have opened the door to change in America. While there are many disagreements with what changes are needed, the fact that changes are needed is widely accepted. Currently we're spending over 17% of our nation's Gross Domestic Product (GDP) on health care, a figure that is expected to double in the next ten years just as it has in the past ten years. Everyone accepts the reality that America cannot afford to spend 1/3 of its entire GDP on health care. Changes must be made and quickly.

My first recommendation is for every American to have the freedom to choose their healthcare. Let the open marketplace of ideas determine what works and what is best. Americans should have the right and the freedom to take responsibility for their own health, including the right to explore options not approved by the American Medical Association and the pharmaceutical industry. Today there is a grassroots effort to establish health freedom as a right of every person but it will take the public speaking up and becoming involved for this movement to succeed. The National Health Freedom Coalition is leading efforts across the country to enact new laws to give Americans the freedom to choose healthcare.

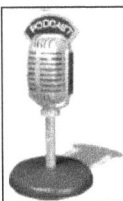

I spoke with attorney Diane Miller, Board Member and Spokesperson for the National Health Freedom Coalition on the current environment around the country and what efforts are underway today at national and local levels.

www.NationalHealthFreedom.org

States have a responsibility to their citizens to reject special interests and lobbyists trying to restrict access to complementary and alternative therapies. I'd like to recommend the Minnesota model which requires only that all practitioners register with the state. They make no attempt to limit who can practice in their state. Like any other business, CAM practitioners should be registered so the state can monitor complaints and take action to protect the public if warranted. Clients should be required to sign an informed consent form acknowledging that practitioners are not practicing medicine and are unlicensed. Clients should be aware of the state's complaint procedure too so there is protection for their citizens but without restricting their access to alternatives.

This Freedom to Choose approach is far different than other states where prevention and restriction from access is the standard. One example would be requiring a massage training and license in order for a CAM practitioner to touch a client in *any* way. Another would be requiring a master's degree in psychology to practice CAM therapies that are as different from traditional psychology as a laser is from a wood fire. Limiting new options for health care only helps to protect the status quo.

Another way to improve healthcare in this country is to change the current financial reward system by insurance companies and the government. Today doctors make more money as specialists treating problems than in preventing them as general practitioners. A general practitioner, the old-fashioned family doctor, can catch problems early which saves everyone money but these doctors earn about $1/3^{rd}$ less than their specialist counterparts. This disparity may explain why other industrialized countries spend far less per patient but get similar or superior results. Today only about $1/3^{rd}$ of the doctors in America are primary care physicians compared to about half in other industrialized countries.

I've referred to the *White House Commission on Complementary and Alternative Medicine Policy, Final Report* (2002) several times. While expressing several concerns they appreciate the challenge and opportunity that CAM presents for our country.

The report understands the need for the federal government to take responsibility for research and promotion of complementary and alternative therapies because of the limited profit potential of these therapies. In America if there isn't a profit incentive there isn't a reason for companies to become involved in complementary and alternative therapies. Whether through changes in the tax code to stimulate private investment or direct government participation, the federal government must take a more active role to capitalize on CAM to improve our nation's health. It will save billions of dollars in our economy so the subject should be a vital part of the national debate on health care.

The federal government needs to become a clearinghouse for accurate, useful and easily accessible information on CAM practices and products. Not every device should have to go through a multi-million-dollar FDA testing process in order for the public to learn about it but the FDA continues to try and regulate every facet of CAM while they fail to regulate tobacco, a product that they know kills hundreds of thousands of people every year but with a powerful lobby and political connections.

To give you an idea of the FDA's priorities, years ago they implemented an "accelerated approval" process for new drugs that show promise in early testing provided additional research was completed. In 2009 the General Accounting Office (GAO) reported that the FDA has never recalled a drug rushed to market this way even though no additional research was done. In some cases more than ten years had elapsed since the drug was put on the market. Is the FDA protecting the public or the profits of drug companies?

While standards of safety are needed it must be recognized that by their very nature many of these therapies and devices do not fit neatly into current classifications. In many cases trying to measure and standardize CAM with our current methodology is like trying to put a square peg into a round hole. New results-based standards and methods are needed and this was clearly noted in the federal report.

CAM advertising practices should be truthful and not misleading to the public but with expanded, legalized definitions and descriptions. For example, terms like Energy Medicine need to be accepted to accommodate the new world of complementary and alternative therapies and technologies. Potential customers should have the right to learn about cutting edge concepts as well as ancient traditions.

While I am extremely cautious by nature about the role of big government in anything, I do accept the report's recommendation for the Department of Health and Human Services to play a vital role in developing consumer access to safe CAM practices. Due to the urgency of the healthcare situation in America the federal government should create a new office of CAM to facilitate the integration of these therapies into the country's healthcare system. However, at this time the

National Center for Complementary and Alternative Medicine has become the center for the federal government's policies on CAM. As one of the 27 institutes of the National Institutes of Health this gives the established medical community much greater influence over government policies on CAM, to the detriment of everyone interested in alternative health options.

There needs to be increased communication between CAM and traditional medicine to improve their abilities to work together. There are tremendous synergies possible by combining the best of both worlds but today it's like *Men Are From Mars and Women Are From Venus*. There is fear and distrust on both sides and not enough being done to bridge the gap. The move towards Integrative Medicine is a positive step in this direction.

There is also a lot of talk today about "results-oriented medicine" as a way to bring complementary and alternative therapies into the big tent of healthcare. Perhaps if doctors accept this concept then they'll be able to open their minds to new possibilities and begin to see new ways to help people heal. If results are what really matter to medicine then CAM has much to offer.

Complementary and alternative healing practitioners also need to change their attitudes because many have a limited perspective. Each technique thinks they need to fight for their fair share of business, even going against other practitioners in the same field. This inability to focus on the "big picture" and cooperate has made it easy for entrenched medical practices and products to dominate the debate over healthcare in America and restrict CAM to the fringes of our society.

Perhaps with more cooperation CAM practitioners can develop a new system to help people discover complementary and alternative therapies. Right now there is no "general practitioner" for CAM as there is in traditional medicine which makes it challenging for people to find their way around the field. People with health problems literally don't know where to begin today which is one of the reasons I decided to write this book.

These are only a few suggestions on how to improve the health and lives of all Americans. For anything to change people are going to have to speak up and take action. Today there are literally legions of companies with a vested interest in maintaining the current high-cost/low reward system supported by highly-paid armies of lobbyists working at every level of government.

Your voice needs to be heard. Talk with your doctor about complementary and alternative therapy options. Ask questions with your insurance company about CAM coverage. Ask questions of your city government. Talk with your state representative. Bring up the issue with your elected federal representatives. In other words, we have to push the envelope if anything is going to change. A rising tide of voices calling for change can sweep in a new era of health and wellness for everyone in America.

About the Author

Like many people I only turned to complementary and alternative therapies when mainstream medicine couldn't help me. (It's amazing how open-minded you become when you're in pain!) I reluctantly began my exploration into this new world following a disappointing visit to The Mayo Clinic. It was hard for me to believe that modern medical science didn't have all of the answers, but I was living proof that their knowledge and technology today has limits.

Being part of the Baby Boomer generation, the group that has changed America at every stage of our life, has its advantages. I knew that the current medical attitude needed to change too. There *had* to be another way to solve this problem, something the doctors weren't telling me. I had reached the point of desperation where I was willing to try, or at least consider, anything. I'm sure many of you can empathize with this feeling.

In one of those wonderful bits of synchronicity in life I read a review of an interesting new book by Bruce Lipton called the *Biology of Belief*. To this day I don't know where I saw it, but I did, and it was the first stepping stone to a new world of hope and health. From Bruce's book I discovered Rob William's PSYCH-K® process and a new way to communicate with my subconscious to discover the real source of some of my health problem.

I took the first PSYCH-K® Basic Workshop and found several tantalizing hints that the source of my health issues was stress caused by the realization that my 20+ year career in supermarket promotions was coming to a close. More than two decades of traveling weekly all across the country had also taken a physical toll.

My health began to improve and so did my outlook on life. After taking the Advanced Workshop I began doing PSYCH-K® with friends. I quickly realized that what was really needed was a better way to educate the public about all of the wonderful complementary and alternative health options that are available today.

The idea for a new, state-of-the-art reference guide to complementary and alternative therapies was born on April 18th, 2006 with a list of just a few processes. As I researched one process I'd discover one or two more I'd never heard of before, so the list just kept growing. Along the way I've had the privilege to speak with many wonderful people. Their support and their words of encouragement made it possible for me to bring this idea to fruition. I hope that you too will find your way to the right process or device to improve your health and your life.

My quest to provide you with the best and most up-to-date information on complementary and alternative therapies continues on our weekly podcast show which launched on July 18th, 2008. On each program I present a 20-minute interview with one of the luminaries in this emerging new world of health and hope.

If you'd like to comment on this book or send your suggestions please visit my website at **www.UnbreakYourHealth.com**

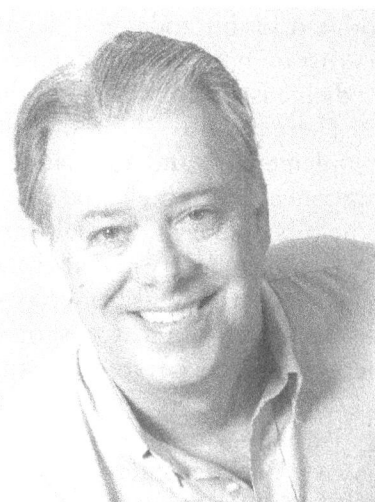

Index

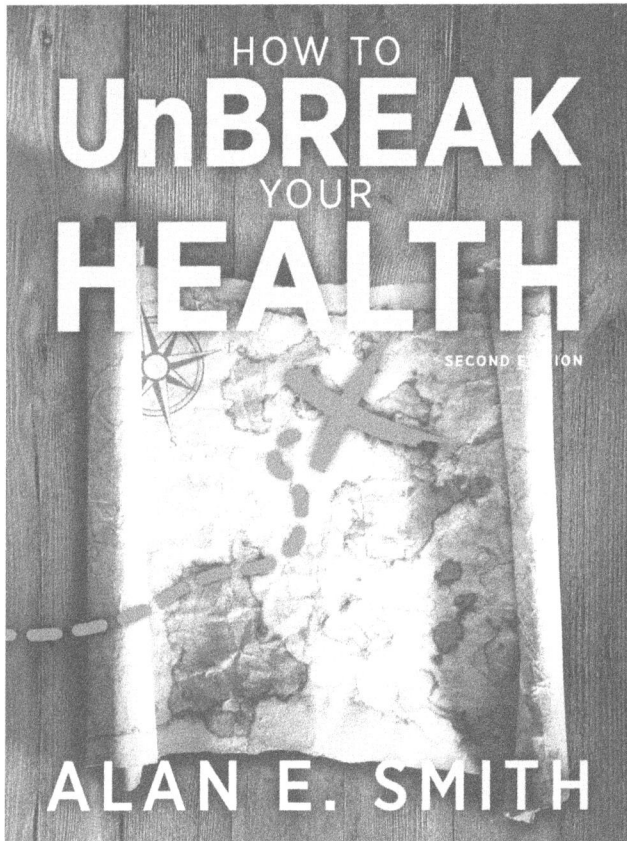

Find better health with your map to the world of complementary and alternative therapies in this comprehensive health and wellness guide for mind, body, and spirit.

Are you sinking into the Quicksand of Pain? Are you stranded in the Mountains of Misery or simply lost in a Forest of Symptoms? Find your way to Hope with the second edition of the award-winning book *How To UnBreak Your Health: Your Map to the World of Complementary and Alternative Therapies*. Discover how your body, mind and energy/spirit can work together to produce better health. Learn how to take charge of your health and find your path to the best health possible.

Trying to figure out where you are with your health problems, where you need to go and the best way to get there? You need a map to find your way around the amazing world of complementary or alternative therapies! Which therapies are right for you and your health problems? Find out in this easy-to-read guide to all of the therapies available outside the drugs-and-surgery world of mainstream medicine. Uncover the latest scientific research that's opening the door to therapies both ancient and modern that are available to help you improve your health.

- Discover health opportunities from Acupuncture to Zen Bodytherapy.
- Find out about the health benefits of Pilates, Yoga, and Massage.
- Learn about devices from Edgar Cayce's Radiac to the newest cold lasers.
- Hear from real people who've experienced these therapies and products.
- Locate free podcasts on the therapies you want to learn more about.

UnBreak Your Health(TM) offers proven healing techniques from the most modern innovations to ancient healing therapies. With 339 new and updated listings in 150 different categories this is the most complete book ever published on complementary and alternative therapies (no diets or supplements). This updated edition again focuses on therapies, systems and devices in the field of complementary, alternative and integrative medicine. Many topics also have accompanying podcast interviews with leaders and innovators in the field.

How to UnBreak Your Health:
Your Map to the World of Complementary and Alternative Therapies, 2nd Edition

ISBN 978-1-61599-042-9

Loving Healing Press

www.ingramcontent.com/pod-product-compliance
Lightning Source LLC
Chambersburg PA
CBHW081419270326
41931CB00015B/3341

* 9 7 8 1 6 1 5 9 9 3 3 3 8 *